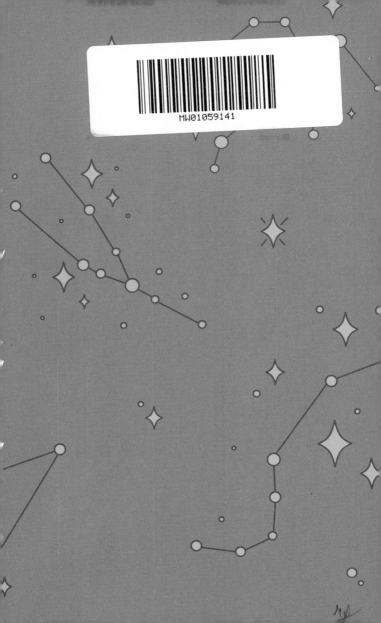

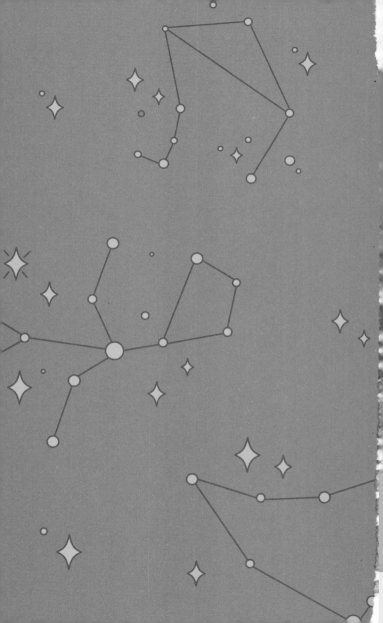

BuzzFeed

JOY *in the* STARS

Self-Care
Astrology for Your
Mind, Body,
and Soul

**BUZZFEED &
BRIANNE HOGAN**

RUNNING PRESS
PHILADELPHIA

Running Press
Hachette Book Group
1290 Avenue of the Americas, New York, NY 10104
www.runningpress.com
@Running_Press

Printed in China

First Edition: September 2021

Published by Running Press, an imprint of Perseus Books, LLC, a subsidiary
of Hachette Book Group, Inc. The Running Press name and logo is a trademark
of the Hachette Book Group.

The publisher is not responsible for websites (or their content) that are
not owned by the publisher.

Interior and cover illustrations by Ivy Tai
Print book cover and interior design by Jason Kayser

Library of Congress Control Number: 2021932461

ISBNs: 978-0-7624-7392-2 (hardcover), 978-0-7624-7391-5 (ebook)

1010

10 9 8 7 6 5 4 3 2 1

Contents

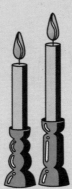

Introduction

Welcome to Your Cosmic
Self-Care Journey

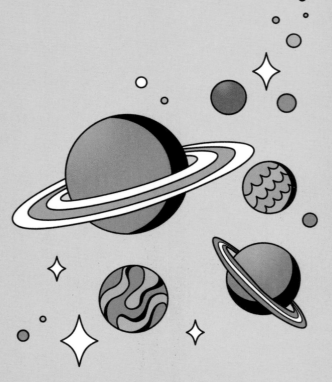

I n order for you to be truly happy, you must love yourself. Why? Well, let's put it this way: when you're flying on an airplane, you're instructed to put on your oxygen mask first before helping others. For some, this might sound crazy—what about your friends and family traveling with you?! But here's the thing: putting on your own oxygen mask first doesn't mean you don't care or love others—it means you can't help others if your own needs aren't first taken care of.

The same is true for life. When we don't look after our needs, we often feel anxious, overworked, lost, unappreciated, or even unloved. As a result, we aren't able to show up for or give others our best selves because we haven't taken the time to tend to our own needs. In order to feel happy, we need to find our ultimate state of well-being. This is where the gift of self-care comes in. We feel our happiest when we feel at ease, in flow, and balanced with who we are in all areas of our lives. In short, holism = happiness.

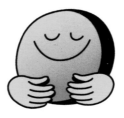

Self-care is the ultimate holistic act. When we implement self-care into our lives, we commit to a routine that nourishes our mental, emotional, spiritual, and physical health. By doing so, we encourage a healthy relationship with ourselves that can help transmit to other areas of our life, including our job and relationships. As with the oxygen mask, we can't give to others what we don't have for ourselves.

Let's be clear: self-care is not just face masks, bubble baths, and drinking wine. It's learning how to better understand and love ourselves so we can take the most soothing actions to help us get through life and ultimately feel like our happiest and best selves. By integrating and looking after all areas of our lives—our mind, body, soul, and mood—we're able to effectively manage stress, maintain a healthy relationship with ourselves and others, and align with what truly serves us while reminding ourselves that our different needs are important, too. This means that not every self-care routine is meant to be the same. We are all unique and will benefit from self-care techniques that align with who we are. This is where the gift of astrology comes in.

Astrology shows us the influence that stars and planets have on our behavior, habits, and character. It's an amazing tool that helps us gain a better understanding of ourselves and how we relate and interact with the world. Through that understanding, astrology also helps us define our healthy—and unhealthy—habits and can help provide insight into what we need to feel balanced, motivated, happy, and healthy.

This is the purpose of this book: using astrology as a guide to *your* ultimate self-care.

How? First, you must know your sun sign. There are 12 zodiac signs, each carrying a certain energy. The vibe that you give off to the world is largely dependent on your sun sign. (There are other factors at play in your birth chart, which is a more comprehensive snapshot of the planets around the sun at the time you were born. Check yours out for a deeper dive into your astrological blueprint.) Understanding your sun sign is usually more than enough information to give you a personal, authentic guide on how to create and cultivate a happy self-care routine that's perfect for you. Those who are a *cusp sign*—someone born toward the end or beginning of a zodiac sign—might feel torn between your sun sign and the following one. In that case, you might want to read both sun signs to glean tips that feel best for your unique energy.

This book is organized by sun signs, starting with Aries, the first sun sign in the zodiac calendar. First, we'll look at the signs in a general sense and how they can help you live your best life. Then, we'll go through four major aspects of your being—mind, body, soul, and mood—to cover the basics of what you need to know for self-care: where you struggle and why, what you need to feel better, and the tools to help you return to feeling happy. From helping you avoid burnout to offering some inspiration for a new workout routine to identifying emotional triggers and soul-soothing tips, the book's ultimate goal is to help you become the best version of yourself with a little help from the stars.

After reading this book, follow up with the companion journal (*Buzzfeed Joy in the Stars Cosmic Journal*) to help you continue on your cosmic self-care journey. With prompts, musings, and even more inspo, you'll use astrology to tune into your authentic and happiest self.

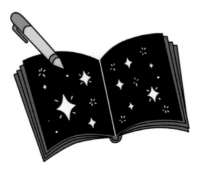

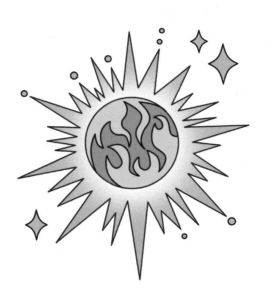

PART 1

THE ZODIAC SIGNS

What Your
Sun Sign Says
About Living Your
Best Life

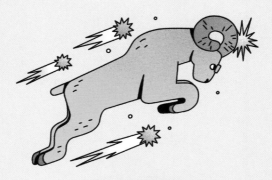

ARIES

MARCH 21–APRIL 20
THE BOSS

At your best, Aries, you lead with serious #boss energy, setting the world aflame with dynamism, assertiveness, and an inspiring self-confidence that ignites the fire within those around you. Ruled by Mars, the planet of action and desire, you're a natural leader and creator. You come alive when you're making things happen in the world. Whether you're working on a side hustle, leading a spin class, or planning an epic vacation with your best friends, you feel at your best when you're busy doing projects that electrify you and bring joy to others.

It's not a secret that you love running the show. There's a reason you have a reputation for being "bossy." Equipped with an acid tongue and impulsive nature, you're quick to point out others' faults and usurp any powerful position à la *Game of Thrones* when you believe others aren't capable of leading as effectively as you could.

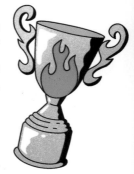

But when you're feeling balanced, Aries, you understand that it's always better to motivate people by example. You do this by staying true to your adventurous, courageous, and playful self. You like to engage in high-octane activities that thrill and push you to the greatest heights, like mountain climbing and weight training. You're always down to actively pursue career advancement opportunities whenever you can so you can be seen and heard as the VIP you know yourself to be. As a fire sign, your electric energy, crystal-clear vision, and dutiful sense of purpose are so hypnotizing that others can't help but flock to your energizing flame. In turn, you inspire them to live to their fullest potential because that's exactly what you do: you visualize what life can look like, and then you go ahead and do the damn thing.

Like the Ram that symbolizes your sign, you charge ahead to conquer any mountains (aka obstacles, delays, annoying people) with a deep-rooted self-assurance and optimism that swiftly place you across any finish line—in first place, of course. Because, let's be real, you don't think any game, trial, or experience is worth playing, doing, or having if you aren't going to somehow "win" at it.

However, your "all work and intense play" mantra makes you an irritable and aggressive soul at times, which is why it's important to take the time to loosen the reins, delegate when need be, and let life flow rather than attempt to force things to happen.

Committing to a self-care routine that works for you, Aries, means understanding that you're a happier human when you see value in being a team player, know how to control your impulsive nature by learning to take a breath, and view your vulnerability not as a sign of weakness but rather as a sign of your enviable strength.

This way, you're able to maintain your magnetic energy so you can continue to put yourself out in the world in your trademark big and bold way—and accomplish even more awesomeness.

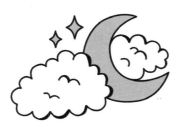

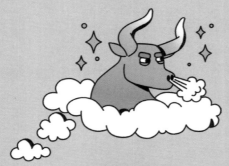

TAURUS

APRIL 20–MAY 20
THE SENSUALIST

When you're at your best, Taurus, you're someone who thoroughly enjoys the pleasures of life because you know pleasure is your birthright. You proudly stop to smell the roses. You savor your food and appreciate art. You dance like no one's watching and always ensure that your OOTD is always fire. You throw Gatsby-like parties for your friends and spend money like the Kardashians. You take the time to love life. While some might confuse your dedication to self-pleasure as hedonistic, at your core, you're a diehard sensualist. As an earth sign, you are deeply inspired by what you see, feel, hear, taste, and touch. And you especially delight in feeling and looking good, #noshame.

You are ruled by the planet Venus, the planet of love and all things beautiful and pleasurable, so when you practice self-care and self-love, you feel like there's nothing you can't do in life. You view yourself as your own work of art and are committed to creating and carving out the next step in your journey that feels most like your true, authentic self: stable, comfortable, and luxurious. Once you focus on a goal that feels right to you, you go after it with all of your bullish gusto.

However, you're in no rush to reach your destination. You have a soft-hearted countenance where time has no meaning. Your pace in life is steady yet secure, and you're nothing if not practical. You don't like to sweat (either literally or metaphorically), so you often refrain from chasing things, people, and opportunities. They'll come when they are ready. While you're extremely loyal and loving to your inner circle, you're also happy to chill on your own. No wonder leisure is your forte. Lazy Sundays were made for you, and you make the most of them without any regrets.

This is probably also why Tauruses are often thought of as slow and unyielding when it comes to making things happen. After all, as your sign dictates, you are inherently bullheaded. As a natural-born creature of habit who loves comfort in every sense of the word, it's easy for you to slack off from your goals and get a little complacent with your daily routine. You're fiercely ambitious and creative, Taurus, but when new ideas and potentially risky opportunities enter your world, your knee-jerk reaction is to freeze and retreat to your security blanket. While you might convince yourself that you're acting out of self-protection, your natural impulse to plod rather than pounce through life often prevents you from moving forward and owning all the powerful parts that exist within you.

By all accounts, a Taurus is a winning fighter. Like the Bull, you're strong AF, and once you decide on something, you won't take no for an answer. By committing to a self-care routine that works for you, Taurus, you will learn that action and change needn't be scary or daunting. You can find comfort in new levels of consciousness and do seemingly hard things to create the beautiful life you deserve and desire.

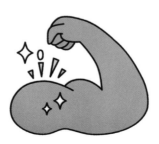

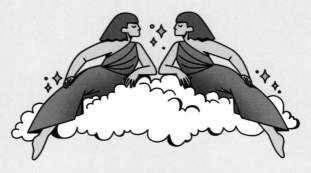

GEMINI

MAY 21–JUNE 20
THE LIFE OF THE PARTY

When you're living your best life, Gemini, you are the life of the party. You're in the zone when you're being your funny, charismatic, and charming self. Ruled by Mercury, the planet of communication, you're blessed with the gift of gab, and you have an electric energy that is utterly magnetic. You are not only able to make small talk with anyone, but you also make small talk riveting (which is a gift in and of itself). Mercury also represents intellect, so you have a keen interest in a wide array of topics, and you never seem to be at a loss for words or information. You're basically like a standup comedian who's also a walking, talking Wikipedia. As an air

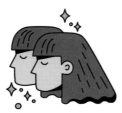

sign, you're inherently inquisitive and eat knowledge for breakfast. You easily become immersed in the latest headlines and find yourself regularly combing through wormholes of random trivia and facts. You see your wit and knowledge as the most coveted tools in your arsenal, which bodes well for you, whether you're dating a new love interest or debating a colleague. Everyone loves this side of you, Gemini, and why wouldn't they? You're the life of the party. You're Amy Schumer!

However, essential to your nature is your duality—you are symbolized by the twins, after all. Which means you're often like two people in one. When you're not amusing people with the funniest meme, you're usually brooding and lost in the tornado swirl that is your thoughts. Air signs are known to be constant thinkers, and when you're feeling off balance, you tend to live in your head. You become judgmental of yourself and others, and your quick wit suddenly transforms into biting criticism, catty gossip, and a brashness that can turn off others. While you enjoy a good debate, when you're not feeling good about yourself, your healthy need for discourse can devolve into you coaxing someone into a toxic competition simply to boost your own ego. You can also find it hard to sit still and have been known to risk self-sabotage to avoid boredom at all costs.

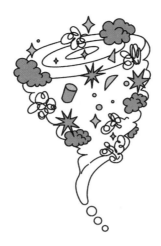

But your polarity is also what makes you unique, Gemini. Your infectious personality and ability to roll with the punches make it easy for you to mingle with a slew of different people while also tackling challenging projects with gusto. Your curiosity for life is enchanting, and you inspire others to learn more about themselves and the world around them—and have fun while doing it. If anything characterizes you, Gemini, it is your gift to turn the ordinary into the extraordinary. Your fun-loving spirit and tenacity to look beyond what is seen allow you to dig deeper, beyond what you think you know to be true.

When it comes to a self-care routine, Gemini, it's key for you to find one that's not only diverse and challenging enough to keep up with your quick mind but also helps ground you so that you can make time to both rest and play.

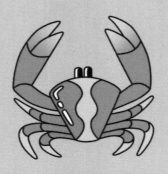

CANCER

JUNE 21–JULY 22
THE NURTURER

When you're living your best life, Cancer, you are the hostess with the most-est. Your life is like one big dinner party: you're indulging your interests—like decorating, cooking, and anything related to hearth and home—and creating community. You're the caregiver of your friend circle, and like a parental figure, you ensure your loved ones are well taken care of. As a water sign, you're naturally sensitive, sensual, and compassionate. You approach your relationships with an open heart and create a feeling of belonging. You're both the nurturer and protector of your inner circle. You gently tend to others' wounds while fiercely guarding them.

Ruled by the moon, which represents feelings and our greatest needs, you're led by your feelings and instincts. This makes you incredibly intuitive and gifted with an A+ in emotional intelligence. You can read a room like a professional aura reader. When you're fully embodying your best self, you trust your gut above facts and figures. You have self-awareness in spades, and you're able to bring out the best in others.

You're a giver, Cancer, which is a beautiful quality but can also create imbalance in your life. You risk overextending yourself when your glass is half empty, and you forget that you're deserving of receiving the same love and generosity you give to others. Symbolized by the Crab, you love creating comfy space within your shell. No wonder you're a homebody! However, retreating into your shell is how you shut yourself off from the world when you feel depleted and disappointed in others. As your helplessness and anxiety increase, you can become, well, a little crabby. While your intense emotions occasionally require you to rest and recharge away from the rest of the world, you can easily become sullen and withdrawn if you don't allow yourself to fully express your needs to others or channel your emotions in a healthy way. The irony is that as much as you're an amazing shoulder to cry on, you have difficulty letting your-

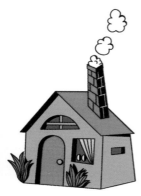

self be vulnerable. You prefer to carry on as if everything's perfect rather than admit your struggles. You hate to think of yourself as a failure in any aspect of your life, and you will keep carrying on with pretense in order to guard yourself. Your protective outer shell makes it tricky for others to break through to you, which can keep people at arm's length. This can cause you internal frustration because you love connecting with others, Cancer.

Your high emotional intelligence allows you to dig deeply into the problems of others and know exactly what to say and how to say it. You're a gifted soothsayer, and others flock to your adroit advice and soothing presence; not to mention, you know how to throw one heck of a dinner party.

An ideal self-care routine for you, Cancer, includes deeply nourishing your emotional and intuitive side while also providing you the grounding tools to create stability and honor your vulnerable heart.

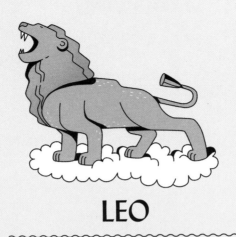

LEO

JULY 23–AUGUST 22
THE SHOWSTOPPER

When you're living your best life, Leo, you command a room like JLo (who shares your sign). You turn heads with your exuberant energy, rockin' body, and fierce confidence. In short, you're a superstar. Ruled by the sun, you've been blessed by the cosmos with a radiant and infectious energy that makes you captivating to watch. A gifted storyteller and performer, you love to be the center of attention. But people don't mind taking a seat and watching you give them the old razzle-dazzle. You have an innate sense to inspire others with your creativity, charm, and cleverness. Represented by the Lion, you're a natural-born leader, and

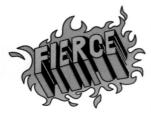

you attract others with your brave and pioneering aura. As a fire element, you're an innate trailblazer. You're enthusiastic and passionate about creating the life you desire, and your fiery vibe motivates others to do the same. They don't want to just watch you—they want to *be* you.

And it's not just because you make life seem so exciting. People adore you for your big, golden heart. One of your best assets is your generous spirit. You love showering loved ones with compliments and gifts. As a proud Lion or Lioness, you're extremely protective of your loved ones and will do whatever it takes to defend them and ensure their needs are being met.

On the flip side, you can also be a bit possessive of your inner circle, and you often feel put out when you don't sense the same loyalty is being returned to you. Although you possess a loud and mighty roar, when you're not feeling like your best self, your ego can be easily bruised. For someone who believes they're destined for greatness, you often seek external validation and approval. You're prone to get caught up with the comparison game and FOMO, which can cause you to chase success at all costs. Your impulsiveness coupled with your ferociousness can make you temperamental and selfish, which, to be honest, Leo, isn't a good look. You might even attempt to fit yourself into a type of prestigious life that seems impressive on the outside but doesn't actually feel authentic to you. While externally it might look like you have everything, you're living a lie.

When it comes to creating a self-care routine that brings out your best self, Leo, focus on the things that bring out your innate confidence while also allowing your kindness and warmth to share equally in the spotlight. It's key for you to realize that your sense of worth comes from within so that you're able to see the world not as your competition but as your community.

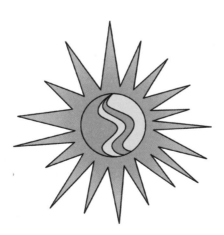

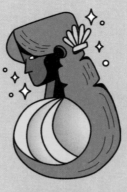

VIRGO

AUGUST 23–SEPTEMBER 22
THE ORGANIZER

Whip smart and brimming with compassion and a need to help, you're living your best life when you're feeling useful to the world at large, Virgo. With Mercury, the planet of communication and intellect, as your ruler, you respect knowledge and information as well as pride yourself on your ability to communicate with others. Blessed with an analytical mind and as a seeker of truth, you enjoy digging deep on all topics, from life's biggest issues, like global warming, to personal problems, like a friend's breakup. Your passion for diving beneath the surface of life is connected to your commitment to personal growth. You understand that humanity is here to grow and evolve and become the best version of themselves, which is why you're so dedicated to being the best possible you that you can be. When you're living a balanced life, you live and abide by rituals that keep you organized and clear to be that superhuman.

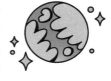

As an earth sign, although you're tough on yourself, your goals come from a grounded and practical place. You understand that practice makes perfect, and you won't give up on something until you know you're perfectly skilled at it and can pull it off like no other, like your sign mate, Beyoncé.

Speaking of goddesses, symbolized by the Virgin, you operate your life based on purity, integrity, and a strict code of ethics. You hold high standards for yourself and others because you believe we are all inherently capable of doing more. Honesty is also important to you. You see it as the glue that holds our lives together. When we are able to be truthful with ourselves and each other, only then can powerful change

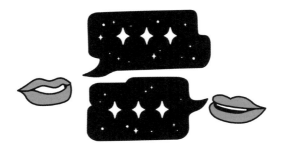

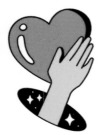

occur. Sometimes you can be a little too honest with others. While it comes from a good place—you need and want to be of service—it can come across as a little harsh.

After all, you do have the most discerning eye of the zodiac—you are basically the living embodiment of the Fab 5. You know what looks good. And if something isn't working, you also know how to change or fix it so that it looks amazing and functions efficiently. This attention to detail encompasses both your professional and personal life as well as your social circle. Everyone knows you have impeccable taste and are an excellent problem solver. Things get a little dicey when you offer your support to your friends in a way that might be viewed as intrusive and self-righteous. Of course, you mean well. You only want your friends to live the life of their dreams—and you want to help them do it. However, it serves you to suspend your judgment of others and to learn that, while you might have high standards for your own life, everyone is entitled to live out their own journeys according to what they deem acceptable.

A self-care routine that works for you, Virgo, is one that emphasizes that you're worthy of everything you desire in life without having to constantly prove yourself. Practice might make perfect, but it's okay if you're not. In fact, people love you for your flaws. It's time for you to see the same!

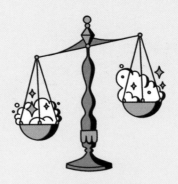

LIBRA

SEPTEMBER 23–OCTOBER 22
THE SOCIAL BUTTERFLY

I f there was a zodiac sign that defined love, Libra, that would be you. You love love, and you love to spread love. When you're living your best life, life is one giant love fest. You feel more energized when you are in the presence of others, especially when you're able to make them feel good. You go out of your way to shower people with gifts and compliments—or even just a flash of your mesmerizing smile. Blessed with the gift of gab and a knack for connecting with all walks of life—not to mention impeccable manners—you enjoy striking up a conversation with just about anyone. You have a deep understanding and

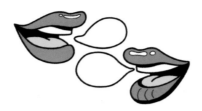

appreciation of what it means to be human, and people feel that when they're within your magnetic energy field. You come alive when you're socializing. You radiate charm and magic, along with an optimistic hope for something bigger and better that's alluring to those who meet you. You love people, yes, but let's be real: you also enjoy being the object of attention and affection. You're hypnotic when you want to be, Libra, and you know what to say and how to say it in order to receive the adoration you crave. So, as much as you love loving on people, you love it when people are loving on you. You're gonna have to face it: you're addicted to love.

It's no surprise, then, that your ruling planet is Venus, the planet of love. You thrive in affectionate and harmonious environments, and you create beauty in all facets of your life. From your wardrobe, to your home, to how you interact with the world around you, everything about you is striking, graceful, and aesthetically pleasing. You take pride in honoring the natural symmetry in life. Ideally, in your world, things always even out for the betterment of everyone. Your egalitarian perspective carries over into your passion for inner balance and equality—as symbolized by the Scales. You believe strongly in justice and fairness as well as the strength and beauty of humanity.

As an air sign, you are naturally diplomatic, and you're disconnected enough from your emotions so you can be nonjudgmental and bring logic and intelligence to a disagreement. You're motivated to bridge gaps, mend bridges, and bring everyone into union and harmony. Naturally, you're the one people seek to solve an argument or conflict. However, you are often so hellbent on finding a mutually beneficial resolution that you are often prone to indecisiveness. You're so scared of making a wrong choice that you can easily end up making no choice at all.

This is why you tend to try to smooth things over as quickly as possible. You'll go for the band-aid or the quick fix in order to maintain the harmony of a relationship. In some worst-case scenarios, this might lead you to enable codependency within

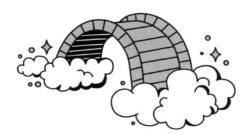

yourself or another. You hate when people dislike you. As a result, you can jump into people-pleasing mode, especially if you're acting out of insecurity and fear.

When it comes to creating and maintaining a self-care routine that works for you, Libra, it's important to implement tools that help you realize how lovable and worthy you are no matter what you do and no matter what anyone else says. Maintaining balance is fine, but not if it's at a disservice to you. Your sweet spot is finding the balance within that springs from self-love and integrity and not external approval or manipulation. You need to seek pleasure and acceptance from yourself first and then seek to create beauty and harmony in the world second.

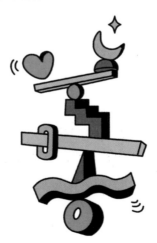

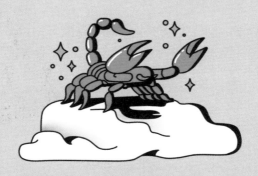

SCORPIO

OCTOBER 23-NOVEMBER 21
THE MYSTERIOUS ONE

W hen you're living your best life, Scorpio, you own the fact that you're the most complex yet alluring zodiac sign. You're independent, curious, and enchanting enough to attract many admirers and friends, yet you're also mysterious and moody enough to keep away any unwanted attention. But that's how you like it.

You enjoy your privacy and secrets. You are deeply possessive of your time and energy. You live life by your own rules, which is why your path is often unconventional and envied by others.

Your unique nature is partly due to being ruled by two planets: Mars—the planet of self-expression and action—gives

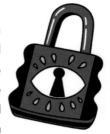

you a passion for life, while Pluto—which represents deep psyche, power, and transformation—allows you to dig deep beneath the surface of it. You are able to see life from a bigger perspective and realize that time on earth is precious. You respect the cycle of life and understand that with endings come new beginnings, and vice versa. You appreciate that with darkness comes light. You're a mystical being who craves to experience life in visceral and exciting ways that confirm you're indeed alive, which also explains why you're known to be the most sexual of the zodiac. Everything and anything has meaning to you, Scorpio. In other words, you're deep AF. You like to make meaningful conversation and connections. You don't take life or relationships for granted, which is why you ensure that whatever you're committing to is something that feels authentically right to you on a rich soul level.

As a water sign, feelings are everything to you. You are the embodiment of the phrase "still waters run deep." You like to feel your way through situations and relationships. You're deeply sensitive, empathetic, and intuitive; you just "know" things. Because you feel everything so profoundly, you require a lot of alone time. A natural homebody, you like privacy and are likely to keep to yourself as a form of self-protection. You know you're a little "out there," and you want to ensure that you feel safe at all times. Even your closest circle might wonder if they really know you. But once you let someone into your inner circle, you're extremely loyal. You don't give up easily on your connections and will do anything to support them—including stinging a few enemies. Symbolized by the Scorpion, you're a fascinating creature to all who meet you, and while you will accept those who you deem worthy, if you're pissed at someone, you won't hesitate to let them know.

Committing to a self-care routine that works for you, Scorpio, means understanding that you're a happier human when you see the value of your emotions and connections, viewing your uniqueness not as a flaw but as a precious gift to share with the world. This way, you're able to maintain your emotional depth while also learning to navigate in a world that often confounds your sensitive nature.

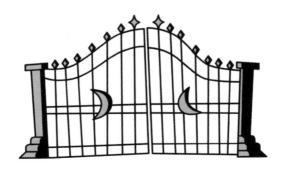

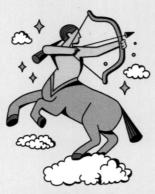

SAGITTARIUS

NOVEMBER 22–DECEMBER 21
THE ADVENTURER

The world is your playground, Sagittarius, when you're in the zone. Your independent, adventurous, and optimistic energy is on full display as you set out to carve a life that is uniquely yours: unpredictable, free, and full of fun. Ruled by Jupiter, the planet of growth, expansion, and good luck, you're the quintessential free spirit who wants to live your life by your own rules. You're infused by wanderlust and curiosity and turned off by routine and inertia. Nine-to-five jobs don't float your boat. You'd rather create your own opportunities and follow your true passions—especially if they allow you the flexibility to work from anywhere in the world. You don't like to be tied down or told what to do. As the aptly named Archer, you're a straight shooter in every sense of the word. You know what you want in life, and you'll do whatever it takes to get it. You not only believe in destiny, but you believe you're destined for greatness. You have a joyful sense of hope and optimism about the world that's infectious—people love to be in your high-vibe energy. Gifted with a knack for storytelling—thanks to your many adventures—and a sharp sense of humor, you know how to charm a crowd. While you love a good joke, you also love engaging people in deep philosophical discussions and debates. Symbolized by the Centaur, the half-human, half-horse creature, you're as connected to the earth as you are to the cosmos. You're keen on exploring both the depths of this earth as well as your own soul and beyond. You are the perfect embodiment of what it means to be both human—always thinking, planning, and wanting to do more—and animalistic—ruled by your instincts and freedom.

If someone tries to rein you in, look out! You won't hesitate to tell them off. You refuse to live like a caged animal. You can be stubborn and indignant, Sagittarius, especially when it comes to protecting your values and perspective. Your happy-go-lucky nature doesn't typically like conflict, but you won't hesitate to put someone in their place if they've offended you. If you're not feeling balanced, your natural self-assuredness and confidence can come off as brash and arrogant, and you'll fight to get your own way—giving in is seldom an option. As a fire sign, your impulsive and passionate spirit is inspiring but can also alienate others if you don't learn how to pick and choose your battles.

But when you're balanced and in your flow, your zest for life and feisty, fun attitude are a delight to witness. Your boldness and commitment to seek "truth" and authenticity is how revolutions are made. At the end of the day, you sincerely want humanity to be better—and you will do anything you can to help.

However, your commitment to conquests can take its toll if you don't slow your roll. Sometimes, you're more effective when you think before you leap and let yourself off the hook from doing amazing things 24/7. It's okay to be a little boring sometimes.

A self-care routine that works for you means understanding that you're a happier human when you no longer live like you have something to prove. You can rest and wait for the next big thing to arrive without chasing the next cheap hit just to make life less boring. You don't have to carry the weight of the world on your shoulders, either. A life can be just as meaningful and interesting if you slow down a bit and trust that all will be taken care of when you take the time to take care of yourself.

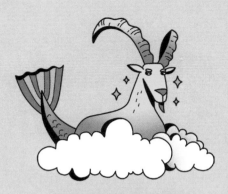

CAPRICORN

DECEMBER 22–JANUARY 19
THE G.O.A.T.

Never mind the boss—when you're in a groove, Capricorn, you're the CEO of your life. A Jeff Bezos. A Michelle Obama. Meaning: you not only get stuff done, but you know how to play the long game to ensure your success lasts a while. You're one of the most clever, most ambitious signs of the zodiac, but unlike an Aries, for example, you're stealth and understated about it. Blame it on your earth element. You're methodical, practical, and patient. You know good things take time, and you're not afraid to wait—and work really hard—for what you really want. You're of the "whatever it takes"

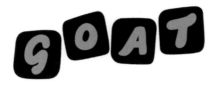

mindset and won't hesitate to put in the blood, sweat, and tears to be the G.O.AT.—the Greatest of All Time.

After all, you are symbolized by the Sea Goat—part goat, part fish. Like the mountain goat, you're willing to take charge and climb mountains to go after what you want. You rely on tenacity and a quiet inner strength to move past obstacles and arrive at your destination, even if it takes you a little longer than most to get there. But that's the thing about you, Capricorn: you can have tunnel vision and be stubborn about what you want and how you think it needs to be done. You're so hell-bent on doing things your way that it's difficult for you to hear others' opinions or to change course. Ruled by Saturn, the planet of organization, discipline, and structure, you're all about following the rules and abiding by a plan. You're great at organizing everything and anything—whether it's a surprise party or a work project—but you're terrible at delegating or taking orders from others. Your seriousness and perfectionism give you a stoic appearance that hides another side of you: your deep sensitivity. After all, you're not a mountain goat—you're a

Sea Goat. The fish side of you represents a well of emotions lurking beneath the surface that you don't often tap into but that you feel at all times.

Saturn is the ruler of patriarchy, and Capricorn is the father of the zodiac. At your heart, you're a traditionalist who believes family is everything. You might keep these feelings close to your chest, but they're evident through your intense loyalty to your friends and family. You're the planner of your group: from get-togethers to group chats, you like keeping your loved ones close to you. But often like a father figure, you're hard on the ones closest to you—as hard as you are on yourself. You abide by a strict order of rules, integrity, and authenticity, and sometimes trying to be the perfect ruler of the roost can be exhausting. Committing to a self-care routine, Capricorn, means acknowledging that you are a happier human when you let your hair down and allow yourself to live a little rather than constantly working. Loosening your grip on the reins of life while remaining true to your grounded and pioneering nature will keep you balanced enough to enjoy the fruits of your labor.

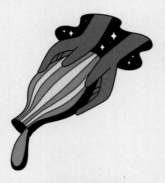

AQUARIUS

JANUARY 20–FEBRUARY 18
THE INNOVATOR

When you're living the best life, Aquarius, you're changing the world. Literally. You're gifted with both the humanitarian vision worthy of a Buddhist and the tech-savvy and innovative mind of a great inventor. Ruled by Uranus, the planet of rebellion, originality, and revolution, you believe in the power of dynamic change and transformation. "Out with the old, in with the new!" is your motto. You want to break things down in order to rebuild, and you're willing to lead the charge. From participating in pep rallies and social movements to creating new systems and ways of being at home and work, you're woke AF.

Your desire for metamorphosis—whether it's for the masses or on a personal level—is mostly rooted in altruism. As indicated by your Water Bearer symbol, which carries water to the parched masses, you genuinely care about the 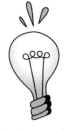 well-being of others. You believe in equality and kindness, and you want everyone, including yourself, to have access to the same resources and opportunities for a better life.

However, your need to shake things up a bit—or a lot—stems from your innate rebelliousness. You don't like to live in a box, and while you might be a rebel with a cause, that doesn't make you any less defiant. You march to the beat of your own drum and fly your freak flag high. If people can't handle it, you have no problem with walking away and doing your own thing.

As an air sign, you intellectualize emotions. You're keen on being an objective observer of life—you want to solve problems and issues with your logic and intellect. While you have many friends and acquaintances from all walks of life, you don't necessarily form close bonds with a lot of people. You believe you have a mission in life, and you don't want anything or anyone to dissuade you from it. You're a true maverick, Aquarius, and you don't want to be tied down. Asking for help or having someone rely on you makes you cagey. You need your personal space and freedom to do you.

But this is why people adore you and what makes you so special, Aquarius. You're the wacky innovator, coming up with different solutions to help make the world a better place. 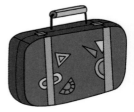 Or the wayward traveler who sees an open road as an adventure and an opportunity for growth. You're the epitome of what it means to be independent, unique, and free while doing what you can to make the world a better place. However, when you're not feeling balanced, your detachment can turn into aloofness as you retreat into your safe space. At the root of your "lone wolf" routine can be a deep sense of insecurity and fear that you won't be accepted for who you are. You know that you're an eccentric, and you can easily feel alienated from the rest of the world. You wonder if you'll ever be enough and can feel so lost that it can develop into you carrying a massive chip on your shoulder.

Committing to a self-care routine that works for you, Aquarius, means understanding that you're a happier human when you see value in a close community and allow your independent nature to be a tool to join together with rather than be set apart from others. Learning to express and access your emotions and ask for help are not signs of weakness but rather another set of tools to add to your already robust résumé.

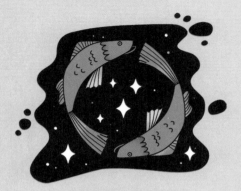

PISCES

FEBRUARY 19-MARCH 20
THE DREAMING ARTIST

As the last sign of the zodiac, when you're living your best life, Pisces, you're the embodiment of all the most amazing qualities of the other signs. You're intuitive, creative, compassionate, and healing. Your powerful imagination coupled with your ability to tap into the deepest of emotions brings an ethereal artistry to everything you do. Even if you're not directly linked to creative endeavors, your life is a work of art. From your fashion choices to how you speak to how you prepare food, you're endowed with an artistic flourish that is beguiling.

As a water sign, you're brimming with a sea of emotion 24/7, which means you're basically a walking sponge for peoples'

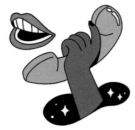

feels. Your extreme empathy allows you to connect with others in a way that enables them to be truly seen and appreciated for who they are, and you intuitively understand how to make people feel good. Whether you're sending a fun text to a friend to boost their day, baking cookies for your coworker's birthday, or being a shoulder to cry on, you enjoy being of service to others. You're the person people call in a crisis because you know exactly what to say and do, and most importantly, you validate their feelings. You know that it's tough to be a human sometimes.

Ruled by Neptune, the planet of dreams, inspiration, spirituality, and illusion, you have an otherworldly, almost angelic quality about you. Naturally intuitive, you feel connected to your soul's truth at such a deep level that you will do anything to honor the visions that you've set forth to bring into reality. Your connection to the divine allows you to understand the beauty of authenticity and vulnerability, and it's your life's mission to cherish and express those parts within you. Your symbol, two entwined Fish, represents the hidden depths and the connection between the conscious and unconscious. Essentially, you believe in bridging the divine with life on earth. You know life is about living according to your soulful purpose. You are allergic to superficiality on any level, which is why you can spend a lot of time in self-reflection, diving deep into who you really are and what you truly have to offer. You're not afraid to look at your shadow side and get down and dirty with some dark truths. But all this woolgathering can make it hard for you to turn your biggest dreams into actionable results. You can get so caught up in asking big questions, fixing yourself, and feeling big feelings that you struggle with grounding yourself. Your big, beautiful ideas can quickly become overwhelming, and you wonder if you're capable of achieving your goals after all.

A self-care routine that would work for you, Pisces, is one that helps you explore your dreams while keeping you tethered to the ground. It's key to realize that you are a happier human when you are in the driver's seat of not only your emotions but also your life. Feeling and dreaming are essential to your well-being and purpose, but doing and acting are how you make your romantic visions happen.

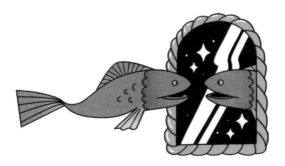

PART 2

MIND
Taking Care
of Yourself Mentally

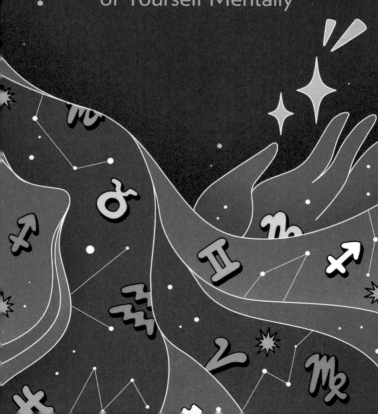

ARIES

~~~~~~~~~~~~~~~~~~~~~~~~~~

A FIERY FRUSTRATED RAM

Nothing upsets your sense of equilibrium more than when you feel bored, Aries. Sitting still is not an option for the intrepid go-getter that you are. Your intense energy craves challenges and adventures, so you believe that life should always be just that: super challenging and always adventurous.

This is why you work on side hustles after your 9-to-5, take it upon yourself to single-handedly plan a thrilling mountain climbing vacation for you and your friends, or sign up for yet another marathon.

It sounds exhausting to most, and while you can certainly wing this roadrunner lifestyle like the high-strung badass you are, here's the thing: if you don't keep a well-balanced schedule, your thirst for being on the go 24/7 will inevitably lead to feelings of overwhelm, frustration, and being tired AF.

So why do it? Because deep down you have an innate need to prove yourself. Self-doubt and negativity can easily plague you, especially when you think you're not where you "should" be or when you haven't received recognition for hard-earned efforts. This explains why

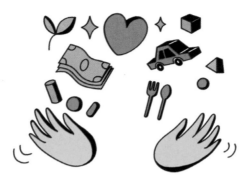

you're the high achiever at work and the problem solver within your social circle. You keep pressing on with your overwhelming schedule and continue to take on extra projects and hobbies because you need to believe you're worthy of all that you desire. You need to feel useful. If you aren't doing something, then what do you *do*? These are the thoughts that weigh on your mind, Aries. However, the need to "do, do, do" is what keeps you in a vicious loop of burnout and frustration. If you don't notice where and how you're expending your mental energy, you'll most likely feel as though you're standing still—and we all know how much you hate standing still. Your bravado and addiction to busy-ness might keep you from doing what's best for your mental health—after all, if anyone can juggle life, you'd like to think it's you—and these are precisely the qualities that can lead you to feeling overwhelmed.

SELF-CARE HABITS
FOR ARIES'S PEACE OF MIND

When it comes to soothing your busy mind, Aries, try to just . . . *chill*. Easier said than done for a rambunctious Ram, but it will help you adapt to a more Zen-like lifestyle. Here are some ideas that will help you connect to your inner Zen master.

Go toward the things that ignite a f*ck yes! You love keeping busy, but when it comes to your mental self-care, it's key to keep your plate filled with only things you're actually passionate about. This includes anything from hobbies to projects to social events. Start saying "no" to the things that you don't really want to do, and say "yes" only to the things that truly inspire and light you up. The ones that make you say "f*ck yes!". Don't say "yes" to anything that doesn't make you feel that way. You'll be implementing boundaries for your precious time and effort, and you'll stick to the things that make the most of your radiance.

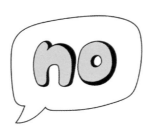

Create downtime in your schedule. You probably spend a lot of your free time brainstorming and conjuring up new plans and projects. But even an ambitious go-getter like yourself must rest, Aries. Commit to creating an hour of downtime that allows you to focus on something less strenuous and more serene. Whether it's reading a fluffy novel or zoning out on Netflix, allow yourself to think about nothing important—just something nice and easy.

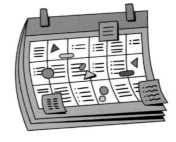

Remember: you're a human being, not a human doing. Whenever your mind is clouded with self-doubt, insecurity, and/or FOMO, remember that you are amazing just for being you. You don't need to "do" anything or accomplish anything to be accepted and loved for who you are. Get into the habit of repeating positive affirmations whenever you start beating yourself up for feeling "less than." Stick them on your bathroom mirror or type them on your phone. Recite them daily. Here are some to get you started: "When I allow myself to slow down, I can be my badass self," "Rest is productive, too," and (here's a good one) "My worth is determined by who I am and not by what I do."

TAURUS

~~~~~~~~~~~~~~~~~~~~~~

TORTURED AND CLUTTERED

The true nature of a Taurus is to happily stroll through life. You prefer ease and flow and spending your day merrily indulging your whims. However, when you're feeling stressed, you approach life in the exact opposite fashion. Life becomes suddenly overwhelming and unmanageable, causing you to overanalyze and criticize your thoughts and actions. As someone who prefers to focus their attention on one thing at a time, you find multitasking impossible when feeling under pressure, and your stubborn nature kicks in, as you want to keep things as familiar and easy as possible. For example, if your boss asks you to take on a new responsibility you're not prepared for, you'll lie awake all night worried that you might get it "wrong" and wonder how you can get out of it. You're one of the hardest workers of the zodiac, but slipping into this cycle of anxiety can keep you from showing up as your best self, Taurus, and causes you to second-guess your worthiness.

When you're feeling imbalanced and insecure, you also have a tendency to attempt to "keep up with the Kardashians" (we all agree they're the new Joneses, right?), and you place a great deal of importance on attaining material possessions and financial security to cover up feelings of self-doubt and "not enough-ness." As life feels more and more stressful, you begin to acquire a ton of clutter not only in your mind but also within your space. While buying new clothes and electronics might initially soothe you, as time goes on, your disorganized home might soon become a place of stress. Clutter is known to affect our anxiety levels, sleep, and ability to focus. It can also trigger coping and avoidance habits, which for you, Taurus, most likely mean snacking on junk food and bingeing on TV shows, shutting yourself off from the rest of the world.

Retreating to what feels safe is your go-to since you are a creature of both habit and comforts. And while there is nothing wrong with knowing when to rest and self-soothe, knowing the intention behind your patterns is key. Are you vegging out in the act of self-care or simply procrastinating what needs to be done? Let's be real: when you're feeling overwhelmed, you're more than a little sluggish. You can be downright avoidant and risk-averse. You prefer routine and stability in your life because change—whether internally or externally—often feels overwhelming to you. This is why it can be so easy for you to feel and stay stuck at times. Your indolence, coupled with your stubborn side, can make your goals sometimes feel far out of reach, leading to anxiety, anger, and a feeling of powerless.

If you don't take the time to question how you're treating yourself mentally, Taurus, you can become overwhelmed with disempowering feelings and thoughts that will push you on the hamster wheel of life, causing you to spin around without any sign of progress as you move deeper into hedonism and anxiety and further away from your grounded and light-hearted self.

SELF-CARE HABITS FOR TAURUS'S PEACE OF MIND

To soothe your anxiety and boost your confidence, Taurus, you must get clear and organized as you take baby steps toward what will help you move forward in life. Remember: taking tiny steps toward change needn't be scary.

Get out of your comfort zone regularly. You might love your comfort, but fear of the unknown can lead to stagnancy and unhappiness. Leaving your comfort zone ramps up your creativity and confidence and helps you to deal with change— and making change. Doing something new doesn't need to be super huge. It can be as simple as taking a new route to work, learning a new skill, or volunteering at one of your favorite causes. You have no idea how awesome you truly are until you venture outside your familiar world.

Commit to a goal—and reward yourself. Getting overwhelmed with multitasking often makes you procrastinate and dig in your heels when it comes to moving forward. One of the best things you can do is choose just one thing you've been putting off from your to-do list and commit to complete that goal within the next week. Get an accountability buddy to keep you focused, and make it fun by rewarding yourself with a treat (we all know how much you love your treats, Taurus!).

"Marie Kondo" your life. When your mind and space are cluttered with unwanted things, the best thing you can do is get clear and organized on what you want to keep and what you want to throw away. A seasonal decluttering of your home is a great tradition to keep your space tidy and in order while simultaneously decreasing your stress level. Even cleaning out your desk drawer or wallet on a regular basis may help you feel better; small accomplishments can go a long way. Mentally, you can empower yourself and stay focused by repeating daily positive affirmations. Try one of these: "I take charge and get things done right now," "I am always supported by life no matter what," and "I believe in myself and my capabilities."

GEMINI

DISTRACTED AND DIZZYING

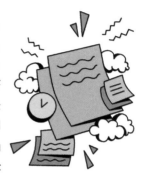

ecause your mind is so quick, on even the best of days, you have trouble concentrating. But when you're not properly taking care of your mental health, your to-do list can become overwhelming, and you might find yourself jumping from one thing to another without finishing anything. As a result, you become frustrated and disappointed with yourself and can find yourself dealing with an endless stack of incomplete tasks.

This would be doubly overwhelming for you, Twin, since you need constant creativity and stimulation. Lackluster jobs, boring assignments, or even the mundane chores of adulting can be mind-numbing experiences for you. As an air sign, your mind and intellect desire titillation 24/7, so you crave spontaneous adventures, new ideas, and creative outlets. Since you despise sitting still and feeling stifled, you could ultimately sabotage yourself by quitting a job or relationship in the name of change.

When you're not focused on one particular topic, Gemini, your kinetic energy becomes frantic. You easily become distracted with each shiny new thing or person that floats into your experience, and your busy mind goes into 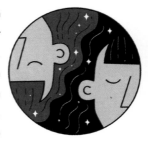 overdrive. Thanks to your home planet, Mercury, the planet of communication, overthinking is something you can fall prey to without even trying. So, when you're stressed, your mind instantly becomes a roller coaster of anxiety-riddled thoughts of needing to say the smartest tidbit or the funniest joke at all times. Basically, you want to be "on" in order to mask your anxiety and insecurity. You place a ton of value on your intellect and ability to charm the pants off those around you. If you're not the most intelligent or charming person in the room, you begin to question your self-worth. And "on" to you typically means being "right," because if there's anything that a Gemini loathes in life it's being wrong.

If you don't take the time to cool your jets and find a safe landing space for your jumbled thoughts and agitated vibe, you can find yourself in a tailspin of incompletion, dissatisfaction, and alienation of those who you hold near and dear.

SELF-CARE HABITS FOR GEMINI'S PEACE OF MIND

When it comes to calming your nervous mind, Gemini, you need a mix of creative self-care ideas that can keep your dual nature entertained while also allowing you to drop into the present moment.

Create a morning routine. While you might not be the biggest fan of regular regimens, implementing a morning routine can help ground your energy at the start of your day, bringing you a sense of peace and calm. Morning routines are known to reduce stress, and you're also less likely to forget something in the morning—something you're prone to do thanks to your whirring mind. A morning routine includes different things for everyone, from setting your schedule to enjoying a quiet moment alone with your coffee, but it primarily helps you start the day on a productive and positive note.

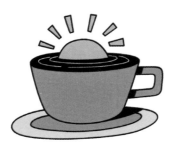

Take yourself on regular artist dates. Using creativity as self-care allows you to support your thirst for knowledge by challenging yourself in new, fun ways. A perfect example of this would be taking yourself out on a regular artist date, which is a solo expedition to explore something creative that interests you. It could include anything from attending a pottery class to photographing the wildlife in your local park. The idea is to do something different—which you love—and give freedom to that creative energy that's bursting from within.

Keep a journal. Gemini is the zodiac sign of the writer, so keeping a journal is great for you. Journaling your thoughts and feelings, especially when you're feeling anxious and triggered, is a beneficial way to empty your busy mind. You can also write down powerful affirmations like: "I will be observant and attentive throughout my entire day," "I am centered and grounded," and "I find fun in the everyday." Bonus: a journal can help you keep track of your projects when you are feeling overwhelmed.

CANCER

~~~~~~~~~~~~~~~~~~~~~~~~~~

A CAUTIOUS
AND CONFUSED CRAB

When you're letting your mind run the show, Cancer, you have a tendency to internalize your problems because you're scared to admit any fault or wrongdoing. On the outside, you like to show that you have everything together—and perfectly coordinated and curated, of course—but at your core, you often believe you have something to prove. This imbalance stems from a deep-rooted fear of failing to live up to life's expectations and can cause you to feel undervalued and unappreciated. Because your natural skills are rooted in the feminine—like being creative and taking care of others—you can often feel like you don't measure up to those who might seem more "successful"

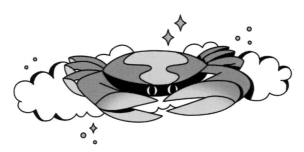

than you. When you're really reeling and in the throes of the comparison game, you might see the world as an entity working against you and secretly seethe with negativity and pessimism. You become confused as to which direction you should move in, and you begin to doubt yourself. You might throw yourself into your work or project with an obsessive need to prove yourself and seek approval from others. Showboating is one of your shadow habits that comes out in full force when you're feeling "less than."

Being a water element and living in your feels make it difficult for you to rationalize your thoughts. When you begin to doubt yourself and/or your ability to cope, you might find yourself going into a spiral that things might never work out for you and that you are categorically and catastrophically stuck. As an intrinsically cautious person who likes their comfort, you find it challenging to take necessary risks to move your life forward. When you're in the depths of despair, it's hard for you to see alternative outcomes that could benefit you. Knowing that you're able to overcome any adversity and refusing to victimize yourself are huge lessons for you, Cancer. But it takes grounding yourself consistently and growing slowly into a new mindset that allows you to step into your empowerment.

The most important task for your mental health is to find and stabilize your inner anchor. So, rather than defer to others' judgment, listen to your natural gifts of intuition and emotional intelligence, and trust yourself to confidently evolve into your happiest, healthiest, and most badass self.

SELF-CARE HABITS FOR CANCER'S PEACE OF MIND

When it comes to soothing your confused mind, Cancer, it's important that you boost your confidence to gain clarity while also recognizing your innate gifts.

Do something that scares you. Each week, venture outside of your shell and instill some inner confidence by doing something that scares you. It could be joining an improv team, talking to a stranger at the grocery store, or speaking up at your business meeting. The more you practice things that feel scary, the less intimidating they become and the more confidence you will have for new challenges.

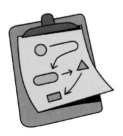 **Make a plan.** If you find you're leading with your feelings on a particularly distressing topic, it's time to lean on your mind. Focus on what you want to create rather than on things out of your control.

When you're feeling confused as to what to do next, it's time to make a plan and stick to it. It will help you feel more in control, keep you organized, and make everything just a little bit simpler. Maybe it's a plan for the day or a business outline. Get clear on what you want, and then make it happen.

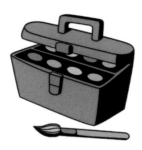

Start a creative hobby. As a Cancer, you're a natural artist. You feel more like your best self when you're pouring your emotions into something creative. Paint. Dance. Put things together. Tear things apart. Do something that is constructive and helps you express yourself while channeling your energy and boosting your confidence.

LEO

COMPETITIVE AND
SELF-CRITICAL

In a perfect world, Leo, you would spend your days creating projects that make you feel alive. You'd be in your element, running the show, and feeling proud that you're making things happen in the world. Pride is a huge source of validation for you, Leo. You not only like to feel good about yourself, but you also want others to be proud of you, too. The truth is that no matter how confident and certain you appear on the outside, Leo, when your sense of self is imbalanced, you're actually dealing with impostor syndrome on the inside. You question whether you have what it takes to achieve your goals or if you're "enough" to be worthy of them. Your self-esteem plummets, and you doubt your greatness.

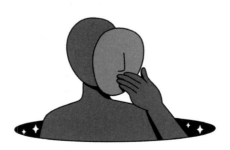

Why would a courageous Lion like you feel this way? Simple: your ego. On a good day, you have an ego that loves being stroked behind the ears. But when you're feeling overwhelmed and confused with the ins and outs of life and, particularly, no life's purpose, your ego lets out a mighty growl. It starts to look outside of yourself and becomes obsessed with what other people are doing. Your ego becomes your own worst critic and convinces you that you're not as successful as others; it brings out the green-eyed monster—jealousy—in full force. Your ruthless competitive streak is on overdrive as you strive to do anything and everything to be back in the spotlight. You might manipulate others to get what you want or resort to sneaky ways, even going behind a friend's back, to seek the attention and praise you crave.

This need to prove yourself also kicks your control freak tendencies into high gear, making it impossible for you to collaborate with others. You fear others taking the credit for

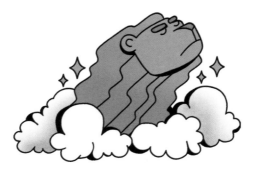

your creative genius or garnering the high acclaim you feel you need to be worthy.

When it comes to expending your mental energy in healthy and happy ways, Leo, it's essential to focus on your own beautiful journey and to enjoy the things that authentically light you up so you don't feel like you're missing out. Don't fear others or being forgotten; instead, switch your mindset to one of abundance—there's enough room at the table for everyone, and even on your worst days, you're still a magnificent beast.

SELF-CARE HABITS FOR LEO'S PEACE OF MIND

When it comes to quieting your critical mind, Leo, it's important to build your confidence and do what you do best: create.

Start a humblebrag file. You're the king/queen of the humblebrag on your best days, but you really need to remember your strengths and talents on your worst days to shake off your impostor syndrome and remember the badass you are. Keep a humblebrag file on hand—in a Word doc, in your phone—that lists all your accomplishments and achievements as a quick reference.

Create for the sake of creating. You're a born storyteller and creator. You feel stifled and anxious when you're not creating something that really jazzes you. So make the time to explore your creativity regularly, and do what authentically moves you. But here's the rub: create for the sake of creating and not for a prized outcome like fame and fortune. This way you'll know you're acting from a place of pure joy rather than jealousy.

Write down a fear list. Comparing yourself to others as well as desiring to be in control are both rooted in fear-based thoughts. You control things or others because you're scared of the consequences if you don't. You fear loss or failure. Remember: fears are nothing but illusions. When you name them—say, by listing them—you're calling out those fears and recognizing that what you're feeling isn't really real.

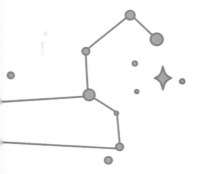

VIRGO

~~~

OVERWORKED AND
OVERTHINKING

Overthinking is your Achilles' heel, Virgo. Your brain never shuts off, and when you haven't given yourself enough mental TLC, you have a hard time letting go and relaxing. You're hard on yourself, Virgo, and your meticulousness can border on obsessive perfectionism. When you're not feeling balanced, you can be overly nitpicky with others and with whatever you're working on, giving a brash voice to your loud inner harsh critic. While your ambitious go-getting nature is admirable, if you don't allow yourself a much-needed break, you can push yourself to complete projects and can easily overwork yourself. You have a hard time saying no. Your ruling planet, Mercury, gives you a steadfast, almost stubborn energy that doesn't allow you to ask for help or to throw in the towel. You think quitting is for losers, even at the risk of your mental health. This is because you equate working with productivity and worth. When you're not working on something that is able to improve some facet of your life, you think you're just wasting time. You must fill in the space of your calendar to feel purposeful and valuable. You

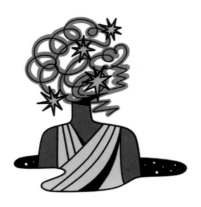

want to succeed and come through as the hard worker that you are—integrity and being true to your word are integral to your foundation—but sometimes this is done at the risk of your health and mood. You can take yourself too seriously, Virgo, and can be a bit of a Debbie Downer.

However, you identify as someone of service. You'll load your plate with projects and offer help to those who you feel need it. Usually, your generosity comes from a good place, but when you're not feeling your best, you can be patronizing and judgmental and act superior. You already have high standards when it comes to those in your life, but when you're not acting from a grounded sense of self, those high standards become almost unreachable and can cause resentment across the board.

It's important for you to remember that work isn't the end-all and be-all of life. Being gentle and flexible with yourself and others is essential for your mental well-being, as it allows you to bring more compassion to your interactions and how you view yourself. Understanding that you are multilayered and respecting that limitations are not flaws will be enormously freeing for you. Don't forget you have another side to you that has a wonderful sense of dry-witted humor and a rich inner world that's creative and artistic. This part of you also needs to be cared for—connecting to your creative side helps you stay grounded and unites you with a more uninhibited side where life doesn't run on such a tight schedule.

SELF-CARE HABITS FOR VIRGO'S PEACE OF MIND

In order to stay balanced and grounded, Virgo, you must rest, rejuvenate, and focus on what can go right—with or without your help.

Think of what can go right. An overthinker often thinks of worst-case scenarios, which just cause you to stay stuck in your head. When you begin to overthink a situation, stop. Instead, visualize what could go right, and keep referring to those thoughts.

Laugh at yourself and have fun. Sometimes you're just too serious, Virgo, which is why your inner critic can be so loud. Take some time to incorporate fun into your life, whether that's doing something creative or watching a funny movie. And most of all, learn to laugh at yourself.

Take a day off. To understand that your inherent worth isn't based on productivity, schedule time for rest, and remember that time off is not time wasted. Practice time off to rest, recharge, and allow yourself to do absolutely nothing. If you're struggling with rest, you might want to refer to these affirmations: "My worth isn't based on my achievements," "I am exactly where I am supposed to be, and I am doing exactly what I am supposed to be doing," and "Today will be what it is. I will be who I am. And there will be beauty in both."

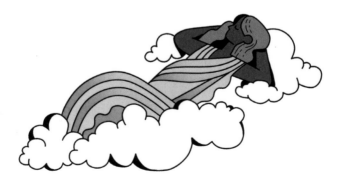

LIBRA

SNEAKY AND STUCK

You understand people, Libra. You love uncovering what makes someone tick. Your curiosity typically comes from a loving place; however, when you're not feeling balanced, you can be manipulative when it comes to unearthing people's motives or Achilles' heels, whether in business or relationships. You want to know how you can hurt someone before they hurt you, how you can get ahead of them and out on top before they beat you to the punch. You'll find various ways, thanks to your charm, to integrate yourself into different situations to grab intel and satisfy your need to win. This habit of yours can be very *Game of Thrones*.

All this conniving and striving comes from a place of fear and control. You love having influence over others, and you despise being forgotten or making a "bad" decision. On a day when you're not feeling good about yourself, you'll act like a sneaky shape-shifter, taking notes and adapting to a situation or a person to elicit the result or response you desire instead of letting things naturally play out.

As the sign of the Scales, you like to weigh things before taking action. You're someone who considers all factors and is a fan of making a pros and cons list. As an air sign, you offer careful and critical thought to any and every topic. Your process is often drawn out as you seek to find a peaceful resolution or harmonious answer that will benefit all parties involved. When you're acting from your anxiety, your decision-making becomes as slow as molasses. It's taxing, exhausting, and confusing to all involved. Your indecision paralyzes you so much that you are desperate for someone else to decide. You'll look to your coworker, partner, or friend to make the choice for you. So, instead of owning up to what you really want, in fear of hurting or offending others, you dissolve into a puddle of powerlessness and consistently come into stalemates in life. Whether it's moving forward with a job, relationship, or anything that needs your self-approval, you can become frustrated with your place in life and feel like you're not moving forward.

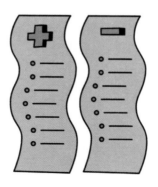

However, as an air sign, you're a big thinker, so you'll "think" your way out of dealing with a crisis in order to avoid pain or any accountability. You'll create complex reasons for not deciding or confronting what needs to be confronted and instead walk away from situations that require your participation. When it comes to your mental health, Libra, it's key for you to remain optimistic and embrace the unknown as you seek the clarity and groundedness you need to make the best decisions for your life.

SELF-CARE HABITS
FOR LIBRA'S PEACE OF MIND

When it comes to soothing your indecisive mind, Libra, you need to balance your indecisive Scales with a sense of positivity and an inner knowing that liberates you.

Think about your great choices. When it comes to finding an effective decision-making strategy, Libra, think about instances in which you made a decision that turned out to be a great choice. How did you feel before making your decision? What helped you come to that conclusion? Make a list and remember those previous feelings and thought processes to help you make future decisions.

Listen to your body. Step out of your logical mind and focus on tapping into your natural gut instinct—aka intuition. By developing a relationship with your intuition, you can instill confidence and develop a better, more trusting relationship with yourself. Start listening to what your body is telling you about certain situations. Develop a rapport with it. If you get an uncomfortable physical feeling when you're trying to decide, pay attention. Do you feel light or heavy? Sick or at peace? Create notes to find a pattern.

Challenge your fear-based thinking. The need to control and manipulate comes from fear. Think about the situations, projects, and/or people you wish to control. Then challenge the fear-based thoughts attached to them. For example, you might think that if you don't complete an assignment perfectly the first time, you'll be fired. Then ask: How likely is that to happen? What evidence supports that? Is it helpful to think that way? If the worst were to happen, how could you support yourself?

SCORPIO

~~~~~~~~~~~~~~~~~~~~~~~~

PROCRASTINATING
AND PRIVATE

When you're not living in emotional equilibrium, Scorpio, your lens on situations can teeter more on the dark and analytical side. You'll turn off your intuitive nature and instead let anxiety run the show. You become obsessed with worst-case scenarios and tread in pessimistic waters to the point that you'll forget to turn on your inner knowingness.

On this path, Scorpio, it's easy for you to begin to question yourself and your beliefs. You'll wonder if what you believe to be true is actually true—or at least "realistic"—by society's standards. After all, you're a bit of a special creature who's always walked to the beat of your own drum. But when you begin to second-guess yourself, instead of owning who you are, you can become consumed with others' expectations and compare your life to others. You see yourself as "too weird," and you wonder if you've gone offtrack from your life's purpose.

When you're not feeling like your best self, you can let envy and jealousy take over. Your passionate and ambitious nature will swerve into competitive, cut-throat territory, and you'll do whatever it takes to get ahead in a game that you didn't ask to play—but one in which you'll want to win anyway. You're a fantastic detective and can dig up stuff to use on others if you feel attacked. However, you can shut down and won't share any thoughts or ideas because you don't trust outside input or advice or you feel too proud to ask. You can also overthink and ruminate on subjects so much that you ultimately don't move forward. You might believe you're considering all your options, but you're actually procrastinating to the point of paralysis.

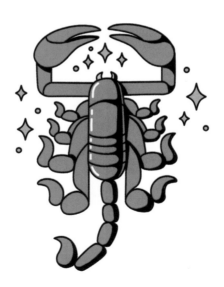

When you're not grounded,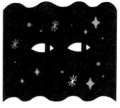
Scorpio, you really do think you're
better off on your own, doing your
thing on your terms. You have
severe tunnel vision on a project—
it's your way or the highway. Once you're fixated on what
you want to make happen and how you're going to do it or
what you think is right, you won't relent. You have a vision
of what you want, and you'll handle it the way you want
to handle it—by yourself. Unrelenting and unyielding, you
don't like being told what to do.

SELF-CARE HABITS FOR
SCORPIO'S PEACE OF MIND

When it comes to soothing your suspicious mind, Scorpio,
you need to build your trust muscle while giving yourself permission to take action in your life.

Focus on your uniqueness. To gain more confidence and
quiet your jealous mind, see your unique traits as strengths, not
as weaknesses—and celebrate them! Be proud of them. Write
them down, and ask yourself why they make you so awesome.
Work on them being your greatest advantage. For example,

honor your depth by knowing it connects you to others and allows you to see things beneath the surface.

Start taking continuous action. Acting on your dreams and goals can be hard for you when you get too lost in thought. Instead of focusing on the outcome, take continuous action daily toward what you want. Every day, keep your momentum going by doing something productive related to your goal. Those small tasks will add up quickly and help you build confidence by seeing progress.

Brainstorm more. When you become rigid with your plans or course of action or find yourself procrastinating, get creative. Brainstorm other alternatives and outcomes. Visualize what else could happen instead of assuming your way is the only way. Write, doodle, and talk it out. Once you realize there are other paths to your goal, you can rest easy and be more flexible with your approach.

SAGITTARIUS

FRUSTRATED AND IMPULSIVE

Nothing upsets you more than when you feel confined, Sagittarius. Feeling trapped ramps up your anxiety. Your independent and audacious energy craves freedom and exciting experiences, which is why you try to create a life that offers you exactly that. Your ideal life is being an entrepreneur or a freelancer who makes your own hours and has the flexibility to travel whenever you want.

When you *don't* live a life of your own design and instead have to work with annoying coworkers in a job that leaves you living for the weekend, you feel restricted and frustrated. You don't like playing by other people's rules—and you probably don't really want to work with others, either, especially if your views differ. You're headstrong in what you believe in, Sagittarius, and quick with the feisty verbiage. When you're fired up, you'll go toe-to-toe with someone in any type of debate or conflict, cutting them down and refusing to allow anyone else to get a word in edgewise. Your insistence on doing everything alone can cause ostracization, which can result in alienation, depression, and mistrust in others.

When you're feeling really restless, you become so irritable you might even go rogue and end up doing what you want with a project or leave work early to get a leg-up on your weekend warrior activities. In the worst-case scenario, you might even ghost your job to break free. Mic drop.

Your quest for freedom comes at a price: you often live life from a place of unpredictability and instability. While that can be thrilling, if you don't keep your mental health in check, you can wind up feeling unfulfilled or unbalanced. You might never know what it means to have a foundation or to feel safe. This will ultimately lead to feelings of overwhelm, worry, and insecurity.

The irony with you, Sagittarius, is that for all your big ideas and plans, without the proper tools in place, you might

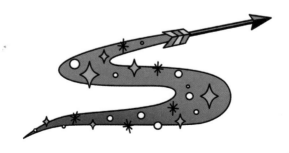

not end up anywhere. Sometimes your bark is bigger than your bite. If you don't feel confident, procrastination will kick in, and you won't finish what you started, emphasizing your worst fear: that you won't amount to anything great.

SELF-CARE HABITS FOR SAGITTARIUS'S PEACE OF MIND

When it comes to soothing your mind, Sag, it will help to find a sense of balance that keeps you grounded yet also allows you to reach for the stars.

Cure your wanderlust. Your itch for travel is hard to scratch and can make you restless. Satisfy your wanderlust by regularly indulging different activities that give you a taste of globe-trotting, whether that's learning a new language, being a tourist in your own city, or cooking new types of cuisine.

Try a creative visualization meditation. When you're feeling restless, you're looking for a means to release your pent-up energy. Meditation helps to regulate the body's stress response to anxiety due to your fear of standing still. Creative visualization is a good example of how to use your imagination to help you create whatever you want to happen in your life. Adding a creative visualization to your meditation practice can help you move closer to your goals by boosting your confidence.

Create some consistency in your life. Adding a bit of consistency into your routine can give you the sense of stability you need to feel well balanced. It needn't be boring. It can be as simple as sticking to the same morning and bedtime routine. By committing to consistency in your life, you prove to yourself that you can create stability, which can anchor your freewheeling ways.

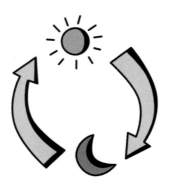

CAPRICORN

STUBBORN AND CONTROLLING

Nothing makes you feel more off-kilter than when you don't feel in control, Capricorn. You like to keep a tight ship with only one captain at the helm—you. You're super ambitious and determined, and you 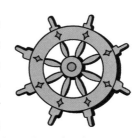 hate to leave anything to chance. After all, you're the one who's taking the lead on new projects and events, working on weekends, and taking classes and workshops to up your game. You have a vision for yourself, and you want to ensure you execute it. You know you can rely on yourself, but you have trouble trusting others to support you or even take part of a plan that you've cautiously and carefully laid out. While you have big plans for your life, you're not much of a risk taker. You prefer to take calculated actions under the false presumption that nothing can rock the boat if you've navigated it on the safest path. This constant need for security and control can easily turn into a high-functioning anxiety. Because you're so focused and pride yourself on being reliable, you may not even realize how off-balanced your mind might be. The fierce discipline that's evident through your steady routines and knack for multitasking can mask how obsessively and intensely you're running your life.

So, what causes you to keep all these plates in the air while burning the midnight oil? What's motivating you to be the next Bill Gates? The fear of failure. Rooted in your DNA is the intense desire to succeed because you think success—the money, the prestige—will bring you the stability and security you crave. You want to feel taken care of, and you want to be able to take care of those you love. Your biggest block is your inability to trust others as well as the Universe to have your back. Your mind can quickly shift to worst-case scenarios—dreams dashed or being backstabbed by others—which drives you to take on more assignments, pick up extra work, or take the lead on projects. Your hustle can easily lead to burnout and frustration, especially if you don't think you're as far ahead as you think you should be. Little do you realize just how incredible you are.

SELF-CARE HABITS FOR CAPRICORN'S PEACE OF MIND

When it comes to soothing your critical mind, Capricorn, you need to self-regulate bursts of anxiety and frustration with grounding tools to help you realize you're imperfectly perfect.

Allow yourself to be a hot mess. Break out of your perfectionism by letting yourself be messy. Maybe it's not doing the dishes one night or not organizing your desk. It could even mean wearing sweats over a suit or not completing your weekly to-do list. Whatever it is, let yourself mess it up and be okay with it. Because it *is* okay.

Reconnect with your body. You can overthink everything when you're in a state of high-functioning anxiety. Connecting with your body can help you make dramatic shifts to your state of mind. Sometimes that means hitting pause and going outside for a 10-minute walk, taking a quick yoga routine, or doing a fun dance break.

See the glass half full. You have trouble letting go because the unknown is scary to you. You don't trust life to work out in your favor without your input and control. Surrender by believing things can be better than you've imagined. Picture your 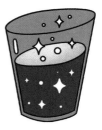 coworker spearheading the project with gusto, or expect your partner to show up for you. Think of what can go right no matter what. Recite the affirmations: "I don't need to sweat the small stuff," "I let go and trust the outcome," and "I trust the process of life."

AQUARIUS

~~~

ANXIOUS AND AGITATED

On one hand, you are a curious, free spirit who thrives on change and making change, Aquarius. On the other hand, you're a logical intellectual in search of continuous mental stimulation. Teetering more on one side than the other is how you find yourself mentally imbalanced.

When you're leaning more on the impulsive rebel side—influenced by your ruling planet, Uranus—your mind is more likely to be scattered and flighty. It's difficult for you to commit to projects, and if you are working on something that you're not passionate about, you might feel "meh" about it and phone it in. It's hard for you to concentrate as you itch for something new and exciting.

This is why you might check out on your responsibilities and spend more time on your hobbies. If you're feeling extra cagey and rebellious, you'll indulge in your fave escapist activities. This might give you temporary relief, but it will inevitably make you feel untethered—and not in the way that makes you feel alive. No, instead you feel uncertain about yourself and your place in the world. Anxiety and worry inevitably follow as you second-guess if you will ever figure out your sh*t.

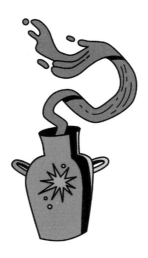

On the other side, as an air sign, you tend to over-intellectualize everything when you're not balanced. Your desire for mental stimulation can get so extreme that you become obsessed with figuring out what makes someone or something tick. You can overanalyze so much that you feel frustrated or cause a situation to flatline—and you can also annoy others in the process. Your excessive need for logic and your inflexibility to consider others' views, including their emotions on a subject, can cause friction. You can definitely dig in your heels when you want, Aquarius, especially if your ego gets involved. Once you believe you're right about something, you cannot be convinced otherwise. Your rigidity can lead to frequent butting of heads and, ultimately, alienation.

If you don't take the time to balance these two sides of your personality in a healthy way, you may find yourself oscillating between two very different extremes without any sure footing and not being able to find any sort of resolution or direction.

SELF-CARE HABITS FOR AQUARIUS'S PEACE OF MIND

When it comes to soothing your disparate mind, Aquarius, it's essential for you to ground yourself in the present for an equal amount of focus and freedom.

Start a gratitude journal. Keeping a gratitude journal is a great way to keep yourself grounded and focused on what you have rather than what you don't have. Sometimes your constant need for freedom and change comes from your lack of attention on what 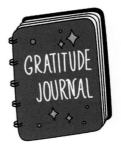 you do have. Focusing on the positive things you have can lower stress, improve your sleep, and help you see how amazing you have it right now.

Get creative. When you're too trapped in your mind and buzzing around with logic, you're not honoring the creative side of your brain. Taking the time to get inspired—whether by drawing, creating a "no bad ideas" brainstorming session, or watching a movie you wouldn't normally watch—keeps your creative channels flowing and allows you to see things from another perspective.

Breathe and affirm. Indulging in escapist tendencies and/or not being focused is a sign that you are not present and are ignoring your natural gifts. When this happens, breathe mindfully—slowly count to three as you inhale and as you exhale—and repeat the mantras "I believe in who I am," "No matter what, I am journeying toward the fullest expression of my truth; it is a valuable road to be on," and "My uniqueness is worth celebrating because it brings something special to the world."

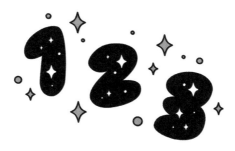

PISCES

~~~~~~~~~~~~~~~~

DISENCHANTED AND
DOUBTFUL

You know you're living an imbalanced life when your head is in the clouds, Pisces. When you're in that place, you would prefer to daydream rather than act on your plans. This typically happens when you're not loving what you're doing. You enjoy being constantly inspired in all that you do, and—let's be real—sometimes that's impossible to do when you're adulting. Not everything is a frothy rom-com, but in your world, that's what you're aiming for, and you check out when life doesn't live up to it. You quickly get distracted from the necessary tasks at hand, whether work projects or chores at home, and next thing you know, you have a stack of papers on your desk and a load of clothes that need to be laundered. Chaos and feelings of overwhelm ensue. In the height of everything, you might make rash decisions based in emotion and not logic, which can cause more of a spiral and conflict with others.

While there's nothing wrong with visualizing your goals and following your heart, Pisces, when you're not taking care of yourself mentally, you tend to get stuck in the "dreaming" and not the "doing" part. Functionality can confound you. Acting can be difficult for you because you tend to doubt which step would be the best. You're scared that your biggest fantasies will remain just that—a fantasy—by taking the wrong step, but you also fear that you don't have what it takes to achieve your goals. You're secretly hard on yourself, and your failures live with you for a long time. You can remain stuck where you are without making any real progress on what you want to create in your life, which leaves you feeling frustrated and self-conscious.

You are a born creator, Pisces, and failing to appreciate or indulge that side of you leads you to feeling stuck and disenchanted with your life. Tapping into your creative side gives you a much-needed outlet for your feelings and ideas, which will only feed into other areas of your life. Honoring the dreamer within is important, but you must realize that

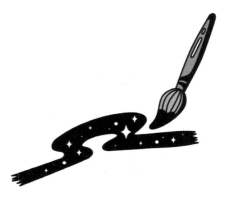

your visions matter most when you're able to shape them into being. You add stress to your life when you fail to meld the poet with the practical.

SELF-CARE HABITS
FOR PISCES'S PEACE OF MIND

When it comes to soothing your distracted and worried mind, Pisces, it's helpful for you to remain in the moment as you explore and tap into your creative self.

Practice mindfulness. Bring your attention back to what you need to do by being mindful. Mindfulness is being fully in the present moment—not in the future or past. Try the A–Z game, in which you run through the alphabet, naming things in your surroundings starting with each letter. It's fun and over time will help you train your mind to be more present.

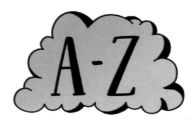

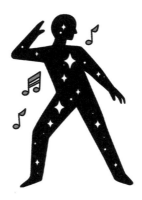

Carve out time for creativity. By nature, you're an artist, Pisces. You need a creative outlet to access your gifts—plus it brings that magical spark to the routine that you crave. Dedicate time to creativity—it can be anything from taking a dance lesson, to drawing, to cooking. Just make sure you love what you're doing and that it speaks to your inner artist.

Stay accountable. Accountability is a great tool to help you bring your dreams into reality. Share your goals with friends and family—having your dreams out in the world makes them feel more real and can light a fire under your butt to act on them. Repeat these affirmations: "I take full responsibility for my life so that I may live my dreams," "Every action I take moves me closer to my dreams," and "I have faith in myself and my abilities."

PART 3

BODY

Nourishing Your Active Body

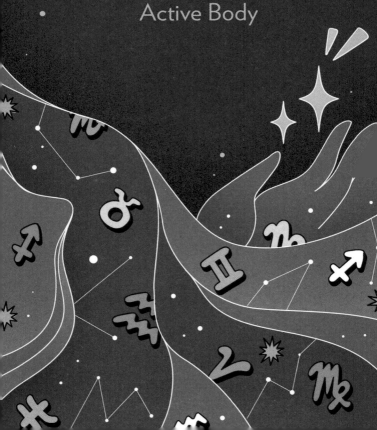

ARIES

~~~~~~

AGGRESSIVE RAM

When you don't create time in your schedule for physical activity, Aries, you get a little cranky. Okay, a lot cranky. Your ambitious nature may keep you glued to your desk, working on various projects; your extroverted side may keep you occupied with various hangouts. However, it's key that you squeeze in some physical activity in that already-busy calendar of yours.

As a fire sign, Aries, you're an adrenaline junkie, which is why it serves you to regularly engage in vigorous physical activities. When you don't have a physical outlet for your intense energy, you're more likely to become irritable. You might find yourself becoming short-tempered with your family or notice that you can't concentrate on your work because you long to just . . . run! After all, your sign is ruled by Mars, the planet of action and aggression. In other words, you embody physical militance. It's also important for you to try physical activities that challenge you mentally, such as indoor rock climbing, paddleboarding, and martial arts. Doing so helps you tap into your innate power and satisfies your competitive side. For you, sweat = success.

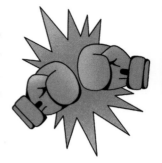

If you don't allow yourself to release that fiery energy in productive (and safe) physical ways, you run the risk of becoming the aggressive Ram, frequently butting heads with people and feeling energetically frustrated.

On the flip side, you tend to overdo it physically, too. You will push yourself to your physical limits by signing up for back-to-back marathons and keeping a strict seven-day gym routine of intense HIIT sessions and boxing. It's crucial to use balance when it comes to nourishing your body. Sometimes that means taking things down a notch and focusing on a more gentle and relaxing physical activity like yoga or a brisk walk. Don't forget your fierce spirit also requires soothing, and your body definitely deserves a break from such intense movement.

SELF-CARE HABITS
FOR ARIES'S ACTIVE BODY

When it comes to taking care of your body, Aries, find balance with an equal share of challenging, competitive activities with calming, grounding ones.

Challenge yourself. A natural risk taker, you come alive when you immerse yourself in challenging physical activities that only reality-star contestants might dare to try: scuba diving, skydiving, windsurfing. Can't skydive on a regular basis? Boxing and weight training are ideal workouts for your ferocious vibe. Engaging in these adrenaline-pumping activities gives you that boost of confidence you crave while also satisfying your need to push yourself above and beyond the same old, same old.

Indulge your competitive spirit. Highly competitive and passionate about winning, it's no wonder you're the zodiac's #1 sports fan and participant. Signing up for competitive races, like the Ironman, or joining a local sports league will give you the exercise you need while also satisfying your desire to compete. It's safe to say you might prefer the role of team captain rather than team player, which is totally cool—as long as you can bite your acidic Aries tongue and aim for positive reinforcement over criticism.

Don't be afraid to slow down. Keep your body and energy in check by implementing slower, more restorative physical activities into your routine. Hot yoga and swimming are active recovery workouts that give you the physical boost you love without pushing your body into overdrive. Remember: remaining in physical balance reduces the risk of overexertion and injury, allowing you to keep putting your best foot forward.

TAURUS

~~~~~~~~~~

SLOTH-LIKE BULL

Let's be real, Taurus, physical activity isn't at the top of your to-do list. In fact, it's probably near the bottom. Moving your body, especially when it involves strenuous activity, isn't your favorite thing to do. You're a slow-and-steady type of person. You only move when you feel inspired to do so, which is why you prefer activities to be nice and easy. Intense drill-like exercises or any hardcore activities tend to make you feel anxious because you don't like to be forced into situations—or body poses for that matter—that don't feel comfortable. In order for you to feel at your best, you need to feel secure. If given the option between curling up with a good book on the couch or indulging in an acrobatic-like sweat session, you'll choose the former.

However, when you don't allow movement in your daily routine, you're prone to feeling listless, insecure, and unfocused. After all, consistent exercise is linked to increased productivity, confidence, and mental clarity. When you don't incorporate regular movement into your routine, your pent-up energy will come out in different—often toxic—ways, including overindulging with snacking, bingeing TV for hours on end, and embodying sloth-like behavior. The more you indulge your inner sloth, the more chore-like moving your body feels and the more enticing "staying in" becomes. As a result, your work and social life might begin to suffer as you feel less engaged and your self-confidence and self-esteem dwindle.

The trick, then, is to find the exercises that speak to your slow-and-steady soul, Taurus. As an earth sign, it serves you to stick to activities that are grounding and nourishing as well as those that require your senses to be totally engaged. The ideal workouts for you are those that don't feel like workouts, such as hiking or yoga. And because you're ruled by Venus, the planet of beauty and grace, you're more likely to enjoy physical activities that make you feel and look graceful, like Barre and Pilates. Steer clear of heavy lifting or excessively sweaty workouts, and instead focus on things that help you feel good from the inside out. This way you'll not only be working out your body and mind; you'll also be developing confidence and learning to love and appreciate yourself.

SELF-CARE HABITS
FOR TAURUS'S ACTIVE BODY

When it comes to nourishing your body, Taurus, finding balance between what feels comfortable and challenging is key to upping your game so that you can remain healthy and happy.

Easy does it. Finding exercises that are easy and low impact are best for you, Taurus. This will help you reduce stress and injury but also build strength and fitness without overdoing it. Activities like Pilates, Barre, and swimming are challenging yet graceful and sensual enough to keep you satisfied. Plus, they're fun enough that you're more likely to keep them as part of your regular routine.

Get outside. As an earth sign who appreciates the sights and smells of your surroundings, getting outdoors often is essential for your well-being. Walking, biking, hiking, and running outside are all perfect examples of workouts that don't feel like exercise because you're too busy enjoying yourself and the fresh air. Exercising outdoors will help you feel

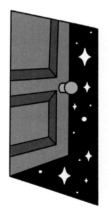

grounded and connected to your best self (while also getting in that much-needed cardio boost).

Cook something new and healthy. You're known for your refined palate, Taurus, and you definitely love to eat. Comfort and junk food are your typical go-tos when you're busy and stressed, which is not only bad for your health but can also get you into a rut. As an antidote, try challenging your kitchen skills and committing to cooking something new and healthy each week. People who eat more home-cooked meals regularly tend to be happier and healthier with higher energy levels—plus, it'll feel great to accomplish something new each week.

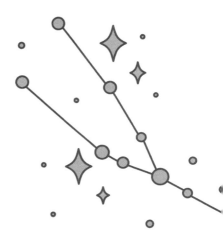

GEMINI

~~~~~~~~~~

TAKEOUT-OBSESSED TWIN

With all that bubbling energy radiating from you, Gemini, one would think you're a beast at the gym. However, nothing could be further from the truth. In fact, you hate exercise—mostly because it requires diligence and consistency, which you struggle with daily. Getting you to commit to a regular workout routine is like pulling teeth. You prefer to live life spontaneously and need a lot of variety to keep you from being bored. When it comes to how you prefer to spend your downtime, as an air sign, you veer toward intellectual pursuits rather than physical exercise. However, taking the time to move your body and finding a physical outlet for your hyperactivity can balance your bouncy energy and improve your focus while also enhancing your health and physical well-being.

Because your mind is often scattered, you tend to eat a lot of takeout and processed food simply because it's quick and easy and doesn't require a lot of thought or preparation. Over time, your fast-food diet will take its toll, causing you to feel sluggish and unable to fully engage with life at the same speed that you're accustomed to.

Your chaotic energy needs a self-care routine that offers both stability and a lot of variety to keep you interested and engaged for the long haul. Ruled by Mercury, the planet of communication and intellect, your ideal exercise program is one that keeps you both physically 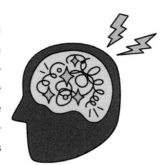 and mentally engaged. You need to feel like you're constantly being mentally stimulated in order to endure the sweaty mess that lies ahead. Community is also a huge deal for you; your need to socialize and chat is as important to your well-being as breathing. Okay, maybe not quite, but in order for you to nourish your body in a way that works for you, implementing a regular routine that engages your mind and body and social life, like joining a team sport, will help you feel good.

SELF-CARE HABITS FOR GEMINI'S ACTIVE BODY

When it comes to taking care of your body, Gemini, consistency, creativity, and community are what will help you stay on track.

Join a sports league. Even if you're not big on sports, joining a league that includes a roster of different athletic activities will satisfy your need both for variety as well as the social butterfly within. It will also help you commit to a regular workout routine that won't feel so stifling.

Implement meal planning and prep. Resolving to eat more nutritious foods takes a great deal of willpower, but implementing a meal plan can help you stay on the right track. While meal planning can seem monotonous at first, see it as a creative challenge (try new combos to mix up your meals each week) as well as a means to help you stay focused and less frazzled.

Hire a personal trainer. Hiring a personal trainer can keep your workouts varied and challenging while also customizing your workouts to what suits your needs. A trainer can keep you accountable and prevent you from flaking out on your exercise commitment. If a personal trainer is too expensive, you can also try using a personal training app (which will also appeal to your love for technology).

CANCER

COZY, COUCH-LOVING CRAB

You take care of others more than yourself, Cancer, so you're busy putting other people's needs before your own. This leaves little time in your schedule for gym time. Not that you particularly mind. You're the homebody of the zodiac—you love being at home more than being anywhere else in the world and find it challenging to leave the house for anything, let alone working out. For you, exercise seems like hard work. Why commit to a taxing sweat session when you can be cozy at home, cooking for and cuddling those you love?

And you certainly do love whipping up good meals. However, due to your yearning for comfort, you're more

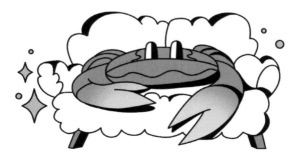

likely to cook foods that are indulgent, which can lead you to feel tired and bloated without any desire to move from the couch. While you might have good intentions to work out, you're also someone who can get looped into past patterning—so if you weren't great at gym class while growing up, you might believe fitness just isn't your thing.

The downside of not exercising means you could pull farther into your shell and isolate yourself even more. Without a physical outlet to channel your energy, you can easily become overwhelmed with your feelings and become more withdrawn.

As a water sign, you prefer to flow. Overly regimented programs don't work with your natural yearning for flexibility and fluidity. You're also someone who needs to follow your intuition. Doing the next big trend isn't going to help you stick to a routine. You need to do something that feels right to you and works for your lifestyle but that also ignites the fire within.

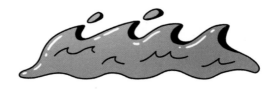

SELF-CARE HABITS
FOR CANCER'S ACTIVE BODY

When it comes to nourishing your body, Cancer, you can help keep your body healthy by connecting to a consistent routine that keeps you connected to yourself.

Commit to home workouts. Since you don't like leaving the house, bring the workout to you. There are a variety of online workout platforms to keep you interested and that offer you the opportunity to do a workout that feels good to you on that particular day. You'll continually challenge your body while never having to leave the comfort of home.

Try low-key watersports. As a water sign, you feel most like yourself when you're near the water. Because you're not a competitive person and prefer peaceful energy in your life, stick to flowy, low-impact exercises like swimming, sailing, and paddle boarding.

Integrate lighter fare in your menu. While it's admirable that you love cooking for yourself and others, consider implementing a plant-based diet or satisfying your sweet tooth on a weekly—not daily—basis to keep you feeling your best.

LEO

~~~~~~~~~~

INSECURE AND INTENSE LION

You love to be the best and look your best, Leo, so sticking to an exercise regimen is typically easy for you. As a fire sign, you're driven to succeed with unwavering passion and enthusiasm, which makes physical exercise a fantastic release for your high energy and something that you actually look forward to. You're always on the lookout for a new challenge or a physical activity that stretches your limits and builds your confidence. Ruled by the sun, you love being the center of attention, which is why you love going to the gym and showing off your skills while also engaging with others.

Exercise becomes toxic, though, when you're working out to prove your worth. It's important to consider why you're up in the gym working on your fitness. Ask yourself, à la Chris Harrison: "Are you doing it for the right reasons?" Insecurities about your body can get the best of you, and you'll go hard at the gym, pushing yourself beyond your limits and doing exercises that you actually despise so you can look like the perfect #fitspo image. When you're feeling imbalanced, you let your ego run the show.

In a similar vein, when you're bit by the competitive bug, you're also unrelenting when it comes to team spirit. You can be such a sore loser that you suck the fun out of what you're doing, and your sportsmanship is traded for showmanship.

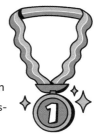

However, being so addicted to your busy social life and career ambitions, you might slack off from working out. While you definitely want to maintain a life outside of the gym, you also don't want to deprioritize exercise, since it helps you utilize your passionate energy in a healthy way.

In order to remain healthy and happy when it comes to nourishing your body, Leo, stay in your creative flow with exercise. Stick to varied workouts that you enjoy and remember to have fun with others and tap into your innate playfulness

SELF-CARE HABITS FOR LEO'S ACTIVE BODY

For your physical well-being, Leo, balance your obsession with looking and being the best by concentrating on what you love about your body. Explore enjoyable activities that connect you with others and your best, fun-loving self.

Take a group fitness class. You feel like your best self when you're working out in a way that challenges you and gets your creative juices flowing while *also* allowing you to socialize. Activities like dance, Zumba, or cycling are perfect for you.

Join a team sport. A team sport is a great way to honor your competitive and social spirit. It's also a good opportunity for you to learn and practice what it's like to collaborate with and support others while moving toward the same goal.

Appreciate your body. A good practice to amp up the self-love and cool down the comparison game, Leo, is to appreciate and acknowledge your body and all that it can do for you and not what it looks like. Keep a top-ten list of things that you like about your body and what it helps you do. You might keep this list near a mirror so you can read the list out loud in front of your reflection and send yourself some love.

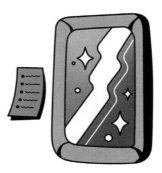

VIRGO

OBSESSED AND SOMBER VIRGIN

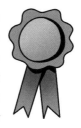

Love her or hate her, you're the Gwyneth Paltrow of the zodiac, Virgo, when it comes to the wellness world. You're obsessed with everything self-care. You understand the most important work you can do in life is the work you do on yourself, which is why you're the first to try the latest fitness and wellness trends. You're faithfully committed to your health and well-being, and because you're ruled by Mercury, the planet of communication and intellect, you want your body to be as sharp and on point as your mind.

However, you can become so obsessed with bettering yourself that it can become toxic. Your body becomes a project, and everything about your well-being becomes results oriented. When you are in this mode, you don't see fitness as something enjoyable or even relaxing but as something you have to do in order to be your best self. You'll work out seven days a week, fervently count your steps, count your macros, and might become so strict with your diet that you find yourself on a destructive path toward a love-hate relationship with your body. You can become very frustrated with yourself if you're not progressing as well as you would like. You can get down on yourself if you skip a workout day or sneak a cookie on your carb-free diet. When you get caught up in this cycle of pushing yourself to complete your goals, fitness becomes yet another place where you're striving to find your value instead of your balance—and overexercise can also lead to stress and injury.

On the opposite end of the spectrum, you're often so busy that you don't take the time to relax or exercise. While it seems counterintuitive, your busy stages are the most crucial time to fit in workouts, since they can be great destressers for you—that is, if you don't take them too seriously. Spontaneity in your workout routine could inject that dose of fun you need to fully let go and feel alive in your body. When it comes to self-care for your body, Virgo, it's important to understand that not everything has to be a project—especially not your body. Engaging your mind while grounding your body can be a great, healthy tool if you find the sweet spot between wanting to better yourself and knowing it's okay to have a little fun.

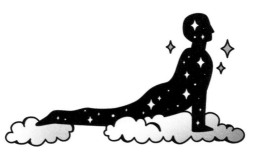

SELF-CARE HABITS FOR VIRGO'S ACTIVE BODY

Self-care for your physical health, Virgo, means viewing your fitness regimen as something pleasant to do rather than a demand. Less pushing, more flowing.

Take a hike. As an earth sign, being outside and connected to nature instantly lifts your mood. Hiking is a great exercise to keep your mind stimulated by taking in the beautiful scenery—you'll forget that you're accomplishing something.

Zen out with yoga. A mind-body connection helps you destress. Regular yoga practice creates mental clarity and calmness, increases body awareness, relieves chronic stress patterns, relaxes the mind, centers attention, and sharpens concentration.

Allow yourself to relax. A healthy lifestyle requires balance. Whether it's taking a day off from hitting the gym or allowing yourself to splurge on some cheese fries, allow yourself to feel no guilt. Remind yourself that sticking to a rigid schedule and routine isn't always in your best interest. It's okay to be spontaneous and make exceptions to your stringent rules. Everything in moderation, right?

LIBRA

CHATTY AND SUPERFICIAL SCALES

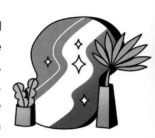

You like to look groomed and polished, Libra, and you love feeling yourself. "Mirror, mirror, who is the fairest one of all?" You, of course! Or at least that's the popular opinion. You're in love with your reflection. Aesthetics are everything to you, Libra, so when it comes to fitness and wellness, you'll put the time in to ensure that your body fits the image that you think looks most pleasing. However, you do have a love-hate relationship with exercise. You're not a huge fan of sweating—it's not exactly "pretty"—which might explain why you're so busy chatting with others in the gym that you might even skip your workout altogether in favor of a gossip session.

As an air sign, though, you're not super pumped about getting pumped anyway. You'd rather spend your spare time learning new things and gaining knowledge. Couple that with your inner social butterfly, and your schedule is often too full of activities and engagements to focus on nourishing your body. You prefer to dance in a club rather than do cardio at the gym.

When you're flitting back and forth from activity to activity, it's easy for you to grab fast food for substance and get by on little sleep. Also, while you're in this "go, go, go" mentality and not resting, you often indulge in sugary treats. Not surprising—a sweet person such as yourself would have a big sweet tooth. Snacking on baked goods is a secret Libra pastime.

Because you thrive in social environments, Libra, focus on enjoying yourself and connecting with your body in fun ways that aren't just about looking good but feeling good, too. You would do well with activities where cooperation and community are at the forefront. Look into workouts that check all your boxes in terms of mind-body balance and aesthetics.

SELF-CARE HABITS FOR LIBRA'S ACTIVE BODY

When it comes to taking care of your body, Libra, balance your flighty and chatty temperament with an equal share of social activities and calming, grounding ones.

Sweat it out in a partner sport. Two heads are better than one in a Libra's world, and you always have more fun around other people. Indulging in a partner-based sport, like tennis or rock climbing, is a good way to move your body while still connecting socially.

Try low-impact exercises. As someone who loves symmetry and beauty and is focused on balance and grace, committing to a low-impact and refined workout—like Barre, Pilates, or calisthenics—is the perfect way to keep your mood lifted and your body toned.

Treat your sweet tooth occasionally. Desserts are delicious, but balance is key when it comes to what we eat. Too much sugar can make you feel tired and cranky and cause inflammation. Save your indulgences for treats once a week— you'll savor them even more.

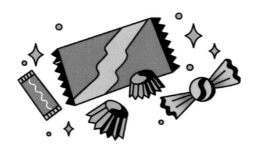

SCORPIO

~~~~~~~~

SENSITIVE AND
ANXIOUS SCORPION

You're intense, Scorpio, so when you don't create time for physical activity in your life, you can feel overwhelmed. Your deep and probing nature can keep you so preoccupied that you aren't able to look up from your work to bother working out. As a water sign, if you're imbalanced, your feelings tend to overwhelm and flood you. Your knee-jerk reaction is to cry it out or insist on being alone to process your emotions. While these are great methods to deal with your sensitivity, a physical activity can also be a fantastic tool to help ground you. Being in your body is good for you, Scorpio. As someone who prefers tactility and textures, when you don't have a physical outlet for your intensity, you're more likely to stay rooted in your mind and fixate and ruminate on issues, topics, and relationships. Anxiety, paranoia, and fear often follow. Allowing yourself to activate that energy in physical ways is natural for you—after all, you are ruled by Mars, the planet of action and aggression. Your introverted side might kill for a night on the couch knee-deep in your feels, but your passionate side longs to express it physically.

With Pluto, the planet of transformation and rebirth, as your other ruler, you're also more likely to stick to an exercise routine that allows you to expand physically and spiritually—that's where you find your true strength.

For you, Scorpio, seeing exercise as a way to tap into a more expansive side of yourself will help you keep evolving as the badass, sexy soul you are.

SELF-CARE HABITS FOR SCORPIO'S ACTIVE BODY

When it comes to taking care of your body, Scorpio, ground your intensity with activities that serve as both a physical and spiritual release.

Kundalini yoga. Kundalini yoga focuses on using your breath to harness energy within you and promote self-awareness through a variety of movements and meditations. It's a powerful practice that simultaneously helps to destress and energize you.

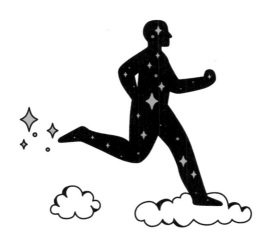

Long-distance running. Running is a fantastic workout that is intense enough for you to release your pent-up, passionate energy. It's great for both your body and mind—solo cardio can be meditative—and you'll love the alone time as you push yourself to new limits (within reason, of course).

Zumba. Zumba is a fun and freeing exercise that will connect you to your body, dropping into your hips and natural rhythm, and helping you get out of your mind. You'll love it for its high-intensity cardio and for its sensuality.

SAGITTARIUS

EXTREME AND EXCESSIVE ARCHER

When you don't create time in your schedule for physical activity, Sagittarius, you can feel contained within your body—and we know how much you hate feeling contained. It leaves you bursting at the seams, dying to break free and move your body.

As a fire sign, you're innately someone who thrives on being on the go. Sitting still isn't an option for you. Couple that with your adventurous energy, and working out your intensity is a must. However, like most people, life can get in the way of going to the gym. You might be traveling so much that it's almost impossible to squeeze in a workout. Or you might be studying a new language or diving so deeply into a new intellectual pursuit that you can't seem to get away from hitting the books to even stretch.

However, when you don't have a physical outlet for your restless energy, you're more likely to become agitated. And the more agitated you become, the more impulsive you're likely to be, which might make you leap headfirst into adrenaline-seeking activities without taking a moment to think, "Wait, is this smart or safe?" You typically act, then think anyway, Sagittarius, but when it comes to your physical safety, you should always take the necessary precautions, including thinking something through before saying yes.

Physical activity is integral to who you are, but with your ruling planet being Jupiter, the planet of expansion and higher learning, it's also important that you seek out activities that challenge you and ask you to grow. Repeating the same workout routine over and over will only bore you. Since you're averse to boredom, you'll end up skipping out on the gym if you know what to expect. You'll try anything once—including death-defying feats. There's nothing wrong with pushing yourself, but not if you're modeling Evel Knievel. It's crucial to balance your need to challenge yourself with keeping yourself safe and to realize that while you disdain rest days, they won't kill you (unlike extreme sports).

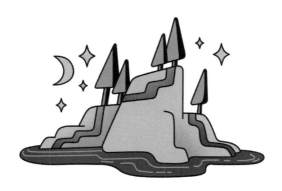

SELF-CARE HABITS FOR SAGITTARIUS'S ACTIVE BODY

When it comes to taking care of your body, balance your impetuous intensity with an equal share of rest.

Mix it up. You need to regularly change up your workouts with a variety of intense activities. Look to HIIT, boxing, and aerobics workouts that release your pent-up energy and keep things challenging and interesting enough for you to keep with them.

Take it outdoors. Whether it's trail running, snowboarding, or windsurfing, a change of scenery coupled with a challenging workout is just what the adrenaline junkie ordered. It'll help satisfy your need to see new places and push yourself to new limits.

Force yourself to rest. A rest day is key for someone like you, who constantly pushes and challenges themselves physically—not to mention someone who is always on the move. A rest day helps replenish your energy while also restoring your muscles so you can go hard on your next workout without taxing your body or risking injury and exhaustion.

CAPRICORN

SPORTY AND STEADFAST SEA GOAT

You're someone who likes to keep moving, Capricorn, because it gives you a sense of purpose. Movement = direction = goal = the point of everything (at least to you, Cap). Sitting still makes you feel lazy, and you hate feeling lazy. You see life as filled with possibilities and things to do—why would anyone waste a moment by not doing anything? Without a healthy exercise routine, you're prone to overdoing yourself and never looking up from your work or latest project.

So, what will motivate you to lace up? A goal. You're a results-oriented person. You probably won't work out just to work out. You need a meaningful driving force behind your routine. Is it to complete (or win) a race? Set a new record for yourself? Lose weight? Gain muscle? You'll get your butt in the gym to train if you're working toward a tangible outcome. Progress is everything to you because it means you're achieving something, and you're all about achievement. You might not be as loud as a fire

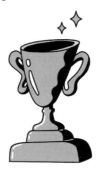

sign about your competitiveness (hello, Sagittarius and Aries), but people shouldn't underestimate you: you're ruthless when it comes to winning. Releasing this intense energy through a physical activity can help channel your aggression in a healthy way—as long as you keep your cutthroat energy to yourself and show up with good sportsmanship. Luckily, you're totally capable of doing that, Cap, since you're an insanely practical and level-headed person. Thanks to your earth element, you have a grounded gravitas to you. But if you're caught up in the rat race, you forget that side of you. Going outdoors and taking the time to be active in nature— whether it's hiking, trail running, or mountain climbing (a nod to your Goat symbol)—is the perfect solution to keeping your physical self-care in check. Bring your being into balance by focusing on rest and letting yourself off the hook with low-impact exercises that are still satisfying.

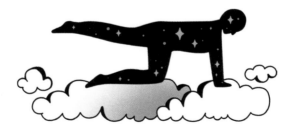

SELF-CARE HABITS FOR CAPRICORN'S ACTIVE BODY

When it comes to taking care of your body, Cap, balance your workaholic tendencies with an equal share of competitive activities and grounding and balancing ones that still make you feel accomplished.

Take it outdoors. As an earth sign, you find balance in nature. Taking your favorite workout to the great outdoors or trying a new exercise is challenging enough for your competitive side while also grounding your energy.

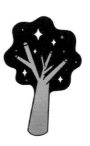

Sweat it out with competitive sports. An ambitious Sea Goat needs sports like marathon running, boxing, soccer, or hockey that show off your talent, skills, strength, and endurance. This boosts your confidence and helps you feel like your best self.

Find some balance. You can go hard on working out and on yourself. Balance your activity angst with some soothing exercises like yoga and Pilates, which will keep you feeling like you're accomplishing something from a grounded place.

AQUARIUS

~~~~~~~~~~

APATHETIC AND EXHAUSTED
WATER BEARER

Creating time for physical activity isn't on the top of your priority list. As an air sign, you're so busy living in your head—thinking about and analyzing your latest work project, strategizing a new plan of action, or simply reading a book or studying—that you don't think about your body. In fact, you can become so engrossed in whatever you're doing that you might not even remember the last time you ate. Eating is an afterthought to you, and planning meals is simply out of the question. Regularly ignoring your diet also means you're more likely to reach for takeout or fast food. If you go for a walk, it might be to help you clear your head; otherwise, you are anything but a gym rat. You already know that doing little physical activity and eating a poor diet are unhealthy habits, but refusing to commit to a healthy body self-care routine runs deeper than that for you, Aquarius. Without properly nourishing your body, your mind will inevitably suffer. You can overthink yourself to the point of no return or, at least, to exhaustion. You'll find yourself running in circles in your mind. What you fail to realize is that a physical release can bring you that "aha" moment you've been searching for.

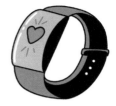

Because you hate routine and feeling obligated to do anything, committing to an exercise regimen or any type of repetitive fitness class, like spinning, is a no-no for you. If you're to engage in any sort of physical self-care, it needs to be quirky, varied, and something that engages both your mind and body. And if it connects to technology or is linked to the latest fad, your interest is definitely piqued. Since you're a sponge of knowledge and information, reading up on fitness and personal training as well as understanding and learning about the body could also be great ways for you to stay motivated.

SELF-CARE HABITS FOR AQUARIUS'S ACTIVE BODY

When it comes to taking care of your body, Aquarius, step out of your pontificating mind and return to being in your body. Engage in activities that feel like *you* so you stay committed.

Invest in a wearable fitness app. With Uranus as your ruling planet, you're interested in technology and change, which is why a wearable fitness app is a perfect solution for you when it comes to working out. It satisfies your curiosity while also challenging you with various exercises and measurements.

Try martial arts. Martial arts—including karate, Brazilian jiu-jitsu, or even kickboxing—are excellent ways for you to stay engaged in your workout with both your body and mind. You'll get an amazing cardio and strength session while challenging yourself mentally, and the workouts are varied enough to keep you coming back.

Plan and prep your meals. It's important to plan your meals, especially when you know you'll be busy. Look at your schedule and think ahead of what you will need to keep satiated. If you're feeling ambitious, take a day—Sunday typically works—to prep and cook your meals and snacks for the week. If you're not feeling that, at least commit to researching the most nutritious delivery and takeout restaurants nearby for healthy meals.

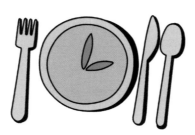

PISCES

UNMOTIVATED
AND INCONSISTENT FISH

You already feel a little floaty and dreamy on the regular, Pisces, but when you don't take time to nourish your body, you're bound to feel disconnected. You're a daydreamer, and when you're not feeling balanced, you might feel overwhelmed, anxious, or have restless nights. You are someone who's naturally sensitive and emotes daily; without a physical release, your emotive state could lead to a state of paralysis. You would easily skip out on the gym to stay home underneath the covers, listening to sad songs and being flooded with feelings without knowing how or what to do in order to feel better. As a water sign, you're built to put emotions first. You'd rather flow or be still than sweat and move.

However, it's important to remember that exercise isn't just an effective way to stay healthy; it's also an awesome grounding tool that returns you to your body and the present moment. Your emotions can sweep you away, disassociating you from your other senses. Ruled by Neptune, with its illusion and lack of clarity, you might find it hard to commit to an exercise routine. You're easily distracted, and you have trouble making decisions, especially when you're not feeling good about yourself. You might sign up for a bunch of classes and attend only once because you second-guess if you made the right choice or if you're even up for the challenge.

Finding the perfect self-care routine for you, Pisces, is easier than you think. All it takes is sticking to what feels good for you and what helps you stay focused and less distracted. You're a lover, not a fighter, so find the activities that allow you to stay fit without being overly aggressive. You need workouts that both soothe your sensitive soul and energize you.

SELF-CARE HABITS
FOR PISCES'S ACTIVE BODY

When it comes to taking care of your body, Pisces, balance your smooshy emotions with activities that ground you and tune into the best parts of you: creative and flowy.

Indulge in noncompetitive water sports. You are a water baby, Pisces. As a water element who is *also* symbolized by the fish, you quite literally take like a fish to water. Participating in noncompetitive water sports, whether swimming or water aerobics, is a great way to move your body so you feel comfortable to you and make you feel confident.

Find creative movement. You're naturally artistic, so finding an exercise that's creative is perfect for you. Attending a class—especially something creative like dance—as opposed to working out solo is also a great idea to keep you from being distracted and keep you focused on what you need to do.

Hire a personal trainer or have an accountability buddy. Since you tend to flip-flop on decisions or might have a hard time following through on commitments, hiring a personal trainer or having an accountability buddy are effective methods to keep you motivated and help you stick to your workout routine. Plus, it'll give you that social aspect that you love.

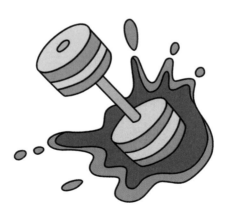

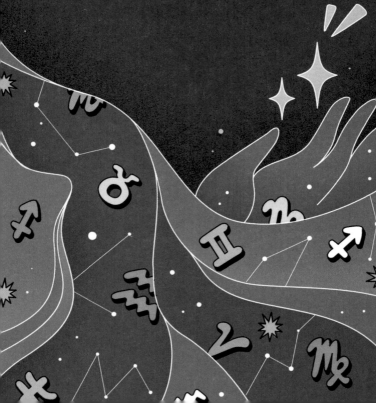

PART 4

SOUL
Tapping Into Your Spiritual Side

ARIES

~~~~~~~~~~~~~~~~

RAM ON A MISSION

As an Aries, sometimes you're just too busy achieving the next goal to focus on what it means to be a soul. You think you ought to be doing something more productive with your time than pondering the meaning of life. This is why you tend to view spirituality as something less esoteric and more practical. You feel most connected to your spirit when you believe you have a mission to fulfill. You like living with purpose, and you enjoy helping guide those around you, whether mentoring a junior colleague, organizing a charity drive, or offering a friend advice. In essence, spirituality is a means for you to be of service to the world. While initiating projects—your forte—is definitely a gift that can keep on giving, it's also crucial for you to know, Aries, that you don't necessarily need to *do* anything to help others. Your infectious enthusiasm for life and whatever new thing you're passionate about is enough for people to take inventory of their own lives and decide that they want what you have. When you're living life from the truth of who you are, others see you as a guiding light and, as a result, start taking action toward their own dreams and goals. You invite others to

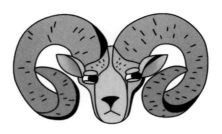

tune into their own courage and lightness by embodying the same, and that's how you find your sacredness.

When you're feeling disconnected from yourself and the world around you, Aries, chances are there are two reasons for that: either you aren't working toward a particular goal that fulfills you and makes you feel like you're making a difference in the world, or you're forgetting that you're a natural beam of light. When you allow your optimistic and inspiring self to shine through despite external circumstances and focus on something that truly ignites your soul, that's how you honor yourself and others and how you bring people to church.

SELF-CARE TOOLS
FOR ARIES'S SPIRITUALITY

Your spirit needs to feel purposeful. Create the time to slow down and calm your blazing energy so you can feel connected to the truth of who you are.

Connect through charity work. Volunteering your time and/or spearheading a project for a cause you care about combines your leadership with a sense of purpose and helps you feel connected to the community. The result? A replenished soul.

Commit to regular acts of kindness. You're a vivacious spirit who loves helping people—even if your intense exterior sometimes hides that. Committing to regular acts of kindness will soften your shield while also connecting you with the universality of our world. Maybe that means taking time out to help guide an intern or doing grocery shopping for an elderly neighbor. Combining grace with action is a surefire way for you to connect with oneness.

Try a walking meditation. Since you're someone who doesn't like to sit still for too long, a walking meditation will satisfy your need to keep moving while also connecting you to your spirit. All it takes is you dropping into the present moment as you walk—sans technology—and focusing on your surroundings rather than what's swirling around in your brain. A wave of calm will come over you, and you'll begin to see how connected you truly are to the world around you.

TAURUS

~~~~~~~~~~

BYE, MATERIAL BULL;
HELLO, DIVINE NONATTACHMENT

Sometimes your desire for earthly possessions keeps you from connecting with something greater than this earth, Taurus. You can become so obsessed with buying beautiful things and keeping yourself feeling as comfortable and luxurious as possible that it's difficult for you to see beyond material attachments. Financial security is also important to you, Taurus; you see it as a means to feel safe and secure in the world. This explains why you can become so fixated on achieving your goals, working hard, and making money that there's little time for you to see the bigger picture. The bigger picture is this, Taurus: your fancy clothes and finery won't make you feel whole. Not even the money in your bank can make you feel deeply connected to the holiness of you. That's because possessions come and go, but the truth of who you are is here to stay. However, when you're feeling disconnected from your soul, it's easy for you to think that having a lot of "stuff" will make you feel good about yourself. You might even think that people only respect and like you based on the amount of prestige and pretty, shiny things you possess. When you're truly obsessed with hedonistic things, you lose sight of the beautiful gifts your soul has to offer. You can end up looking for completeness through a relentless and anxiety-riddled pursuit of what you think will make you happy.

Your true nature, Taurus, is someone who's deeply connected to the world and those around you. As an earth sign, you have a great appreciation for nature, and people adore being in your soothing and generous spirit, thanks to your ruling planet, Venus. Connecting to your soul means allowing yourself to see how truly lovable you are without attaching love to a designer label or any other thing, and it means remembering that your oneness begins with being in nature. Moving away from seeking pleasure and safety from the external is your path to coming home to your true self and to a world beyond the physical. When you recognize that what makes you feel whole and safe is actually *you*, Taurus, you can finally let go and be free.

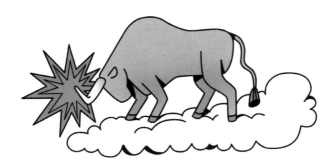

SELF-CARE TOOLS
FOR TAURUS'S SPIRITUALITY

In order to connect to your soul, Taurus, you need to feel at ease and at peace while experiencing the things that are most enjoyable to the Bull.

Practice nonattachment with a gratitude journal. Starting a gratitude journal is a great way to let go of your attachment to material comforts. When you start to notice what you already have in your life—everything from good friends to a beautiful sunrise—you're able to appreciate it more and recognize that you actually have all that you need. Over time, you won't seek fulfillment from external things but from what is already yours, including things within. Even just giving thanks for five things in your life each day makes a difference.

See the sacred outdoors. You inherently find nature healing. As an earth sign, being outdoors naturally grounds you and helps put life in perspective for you. Regularly removing yourself from the hustle and bustle of our modern-day consumer culture and getting back to the great outdoors will help you discover your own true nature and connect to a deep level of peace and clarity. As someone who enjoys ease and flow, taking time to connect with the soothing rhythm of Mother Nature is a great way for you to tune in to your spirit.

Mindful eating. You love food, which is why you might want to take your spiritual practice to your meals. Eating mindfully—taking the time to really taste, smell, and swallow your food—brings you back to the present moment while engaging your senses. Mindful eating allows you to connect more with the food you eat and can also help you make more nourishing and healthy choices. Dining becomes less utilitarian and indulgent and more like a sacred soulful ritual.

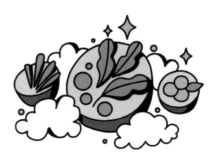

GEMINI

~~~~~~~~~~~~~

LEARNING TO LOVE THE STILLNESS
AND SOUND OF SILENCE

As an air sign, Gemini, you're naturally drawn to questioning the world around you. Your natural thirst for knowledge has probably led you to explore different topics and philosophies on religion and spirituality. Diving deep into your soul, however, requires lots of solo time, focus, and the implementation of a spiritual ritual of some kind, which can be a bit difficult for you to commit to. As a social creature, you have a hard time finding downtime. There are just too many places to go and people to see! While connecting with people and keeping busy make you feel good, not taking the time to recharge and connect with your soul can make you feel a little cranky and disconnected from the bigger picture. The thing is, Gemini, you're self-aware enough to know that there's more than meets the eye in the Universe, and this knowledge thrills you. Homing in on that excitement is your special sauce and helps you tap into the deeper side of yourself. While one-half of you longs to laugh and have fun, the other half of you revels in critical thinking and learning more about other dimensions that could bring you closer to a new level of consciousness. After all, discovering more about the world and heightening your understanding of it is your jam. The rub is, of course, how much time and attention you're willing to spend on your soul. As someone who has trouble being in the moment and concentrating on one thing at a time, it takes work for you to be still and listen to your inner voice. However, the work of spirit is ever constant and ever evolving, and doing things we aren't comfortable with is, ultimately, the work of the soul. When you're able to lean into the discomfort and make small intentional actions toward listening to your spirit, you'll find that the world opens up for you in new and expansive ways.

SELF-CARE TOOLS
FOR GEMINI'S SPIRITUALITY

In order for you to feel connected to your soul, you need to slow your busy mind and drop down into the truth of who you are, distraction-free.

Keep a gratitude list. It's easy for you to get caught up in new ideas, events, and people. Sometimes it's hard for you to stay present and acknowledge the smaller blessings in your life. Keeping a daily gratitude list will help you focus on what's going well for you and shows you evidence of the magic around you.

Make alone time a regular thing. You long for the company of others so much, Gemini, that you forget how powerful your own presence is. Making the time to be alone is a precious gift that you can give yourself. It allows you to recharge and tune into yourself free of distraction and other people's energy. This could include anything from going for a walk in a park to quietly reading a book alone. Just make sure whatever you're doing requires some solo stillness.

Practice mindfulness during the day. Mindfulness is simply slowing down and observing the physical and emotional sensations you are experiencing in the moment—this could be anything from taking a walk to eating your food. Continuously practicing mindfulness throughout your day, whether you're on the bus or at your desk, can help you stay connected to the world around you while improving your ability to focus and stay present.

CANCER

COMPASSIONATE COSMIC CRAB

Cancer, you become disconnected from your spirituality whenever you become too focused on your feelings and become overwhelmed with your life's conflicts or drama. When you're drowning in a sea of emotions, you fail to see the natural spiritual gifts you possess. You're naturally intuitive and connected to the cosmos—you are ruled by the moon, after all—but when you spend too much time denying your natural gift and trying to rationalize your feelings or negating your sixth sense, you do yourself a disservice. Your inner voice and its power connect you to the divine. Lean into your intuitive side, and let it guide you to your soul's truth.

When you're too wrapped up in the opinions of others or have trouble connecting with your true spirit, you can become judgmental and shut down your heart. And your heart is the most blessed gift that you have to share with the world. You're one of the most compassionate and nurturing signs of the zodiac, with the power to selflessly create beautiful connec-

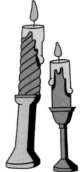

tions on earth. When you separate yourself from others, you can forget that your open heart can help serve others in powerful ways. When we selflessly connect to people through our empathy and sympathy, we allow a sense of an otherworldly presence to take over and reaffirm our faith in each other. Allow yourself to see the suffering in the world and know that simply showing up as your true self is more than enough to help heal the world and experience heaven on earth.

SELF-CARE TOOLS FOR CANCER'S SPIRITUALITY

You, Cancer, need to celebrate your innate intuition while also showing up for others in your community to help you connect to a world outside of yourself.

Commit to a lunar practice. Since you're ruled by the moon, commit to a ritual on any Monday (otherwise known as Moon Day) and on new and full moon days to tune in to your spiritual energies. Meditate, set an intention for the week, and create some moon water (simply leave a glass or container of water outdoors to charge under the moonlight) to further develop your intuition and connection to the Universe.

Give back to the community. You have such a loving and caring nature, but you tend to be protective about how much time and energy you spend on others, especially when you're feeling disconnected from yourself and the world around you. Get out of your head and closer to your true nature by volunteering somewhere that brings out your nurturing side, like an animal shelter or soup kitchen.

Tap into your inner voice regularly. Your intuition is your superpower when it comes to connecting to your soul. It requires regular training like any other modality, so keep it sharp with automatic writing and journaling, a practice in which you ask your intuition for guidance and insight and then write down the guidance that you receive.

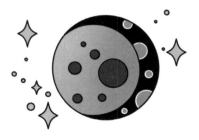

LEO

————————————————————

LIGHT- AND LOVE-FILLED LION

As a Leo, you're concerned with external excitement and approval rather than seeking fulfillment internally, so you have trouble fitting soulful inventory into your busy social calendar. You think you should be creating exciting projects and experiencing life in big and beautiful ways rather than sitting still and going within. When you're not connecting with yourself on a deep level, Leo, it's typically because you're more interested in the desires of your ego and, thus, see spirituality as unsatisfying and boring. You're too busy chasing lofty goals and expanding your social circle rather than seeking solace and value in a power that's bigger than applause. You become addicted to the spotlight and not the light from within. You'll go out of your way to get what you want, even if at the cost of others.

You might even become interested in spirituality on a superficial level. You'll drink green juice, commit to a meditation practice, and buy crystals for the sake of appearances—and the likes on social media. You'll dip your toe into spirituality but only so deep that it sustains your interest and so you can use it as a fascinating sound bite for one of your many social engagements.

What you fail to realize, Leo, is that with the Sun as your ruler, when you're being you in the most authentic and heart-filled way, you are connecting to spirit. You are the embodiment of love and light 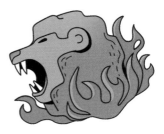 when you get out of your mind and drop into your naturally big heart. When you're stripped of your need to entertain and impress others, you are the most magnanimous and generous soul in the room. Your unique beauty, Leo, is your strong sense of who you are, your natural expressive self, and how you tend to help the underdog when the going gets tough. It needn't be hard—your innate gifts can help you connect to your soul. When you begin to see that inner exploration is just as valid as—if not more valid than—outer exploration and that people love you not for your success and accolades but for the loving being you truly are, then you'll see the light that you've possessed all along.

SELF-CARE TOOLS FOR LEO'S SPIRITUALITY

For your spirit to grow and evolve, Leo, it's important to implement regular selfless practices to further connect you with the world around you and remind yourself just how kind and loving you really are.

Do small, kind things often. Whether it's treating a stranger to a coffee or buying groceries for an elderly neighbor, small acts of service help you work toward selflessness, not self-involvement. This practice will connect you to your natural loving soul when you remember that generosity is how we honor and express human value and our interconnectedness to each other.

Practice chanting. Chanting is not only a performative ritual that will speak to your need to express; it's also a great way to connect with your inner spirit. Chanting is a free-flowing creative spiritual practice that helps you let go and connects you to the present moment as well as a power outside of yourself. You might want to start simply by repeating, "Om" and feeling its resonance throughout your body.

Donate your time and/or money—anonymously. A great way to show up in your integrity is to do something admirable—like donating your time to a favorite charity or regularly donating money to a beloved cause—anonymously. This way you connect wholeheartedly to helpful acts of service without doing it for a round of applause. (Don't worry—the Universe is probably giving you a fist bump anyway.)

VIRGO

DIVINE AND DEDICATED

You naturally desire to be of service, Virgo, and you consistently make yourself available to help others. Symbolized by the Virgin, you're inherently altruistic. You find meaning in being spiritual, and you've dedicated yourself to living your truth from the inside out. However, when you're not living fully in your integrity, you can come across as holier-than-thou. You may view your spiritual quest as more of an inspirational example to others rather than something that benefits the greater good.

Like many of your projects, your spirituality can become just another task on your to-do list. Instead of surrendering to it, you overanalyze it. While being committed to digging deep into life's biggest truths is powerful stuff, if you're feeling off balance, you can also get caught up in the whys of the world. Because you're ruled by Mercury, the planet of communication and intellect, you can be too logical and scientifically minded for your own good. Since you can't help but be a perfectionist, you have a hard time allowing life to be spontaneous and magical. You seek to control the outcomes of life rather than letting them unfold. As much as you want to believe, it's difficult for you to surrender to a force bigger than yourself. Believing that you're protected and supported is scary for you; it's hard for you to fully trust in another—whether it's your community or the divine.

But spirituality is part of who you are, Virgo—you are meant to live from your soul. As an earth sign, you are intricately connected to the world around you. It's easy for you to feel at peace in nature and see the Universe as an expansion of love that encompasses us all. It will help you to find a spiritual practice that's yours and yours alone and that feels personal to you. It's also important for you to spend time alone for personal reflection—and to do this when you're not seeking to fix yourself but to just be with yourself. Perhaps the biggest piece of your soulful self-care is letting go of perfection and control, Virgo, and knowing you're enough as you are. Allow life—and others—to show up for you.

SELF-CARE TOOLS FOR VIRGO'S SPIRITUALITY

You need to feel productive and of service, but you also need a sense of groundedness and faith in something that's bigger than yourself in the great beyond. You need to tap into your spirit to remember you are taken care of and supported.

Develop a regular spiritual practice within your schedule. Routines and organization are your jam, Virgo. Implementing a spiritual practice into your day (like a 15-minute journaling ritual in the morning while you drink your coffee) will help you stick to regularly excavating your soul, keeping you feeling connected and at peace.

Sit outside and meditate. Meditating outdoors is a beneficial way to connect you to both the great outdoors and the present moment in a grounded and nourishing way. Meditating outdoors activates our senses, allowing your practice to come alive and to captivate you. It allows you a time of solace that is truly about you and Mother Nature.

Read a sacred text. You're all about knowledge and learning more about the world, Virgo, so dedicating some time to reading a sacred text every week will connect you to the intellect that your mind needs and the soulful truths that your spirit craves.

LIBRA

COMMUNITY AND SELF-LOVE
FOR THE SCALES

As a Libra, you can be so busy with your packed schedule that you have little time to think about your soul's purpose, which is ironic because you have one of the most loving souls on the planet. You care about people, and you believe in the goodness of the human race. You're someone who's regularly tuned in to the beauty of life—whether it's admiring art or Mother Nature. This, in essence, is connecting to your spirit. However, the everyday noise of modern life often drowns out that deep appreciation of all that surrounds you. The busier you are, Libra, the more you need those moments to connect to your spirit, but the less likely that you'll allow yourself the time to do it.

You're more likely to seek oneness from the approval of your friends and family rather than go within. When you're disconnected from yourself, you ask incessantly for the input of others and remain indecisive about your life's choices out of fear and judgment. The thing is that being around others gives you a sense of purpose. You like connecting with others, and you enjoy doing things for those you care about. While community and kindness are definitely tenets of spirituality, self-actualization comes from allowing yourself to give the same type of love and generosity you so freely give to others. If you're constantly giving gifts and doing favors for others in order to feel fulfilled and loved, you're preventing yourself from receiving goodwill and love from yourself and the Universe.

You need to trust that you are lovable, Libra, just as you are—no strings attached. Your ability to bring people together and make them feel good is a blessing, but the messaging only gets through when your love comes from a clear channel. You need to give and expect nothing in return while also allowing yourself to receive. You're doing your soul's work when you realize you have nothing to prove and that you possess all the tools, knowledge, and love you need from within. Be still, and listen.

SELF-CARE TOOLS
FOR LIBRA'S SPIRITUALITY

Your Libra spirit needs to feel connected to others while also connecting to your inner self and inner knowing so you can find your true center.

Meditate. A daily meditation practice will help you surrender to the present moment, connect with your authentic soul in total solitude, and release any fears that keep you clinging to what no longer serves you.

Go to a place of worship—or a spiritual gathering. Community is everything to you, Libra, and you are gifted with bringing people together, including those of different faiths. Attending a regular religious or spiritual ritual and event or hosting one yourself will lighten your spirit and keep you connected to the world around you.

Connect with your spirit through writing. Free writing is a powerful way to connect with your inner voice and spirit. Take a quiet moment for yourself and allow yourself to write from a very still place. In this way, you are connecting to your inner guide, who knows you best. You'll feel guided and protected.

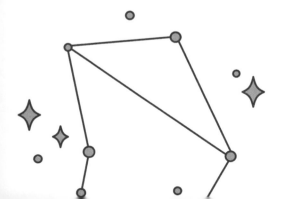

SCORPIO

SOULFUL SCORPION

You're a big believer in otherworldly experiences, Scorpio. You know the truth is out there. With your Mars and Pluto planet-ruling duo, you're intense about your dogma. You see life as a transformational experience. Why else are we here? Your imbalance with spirituality comes when you're living life more esoterically and, dare I say it, acting preachy? You are known to stand up on your soapbox and preach to others about your belief system. You might view yourself as a spiritual guru in your circle of friends, and you enjoy spreading your wisdom and spiritual knowledge to them in order to help "heal" and fix their lives. What you fail to realize is that most people learn by example. You need to walk your talk, Scorpio, which isn't something you always do. The thing is, Scorpio, you know what you believe in. You have a clear sense of how you think the Universe and soul work on a very philosophical and deep level. But sometimes you have a hard time when it comes to putting your work into practice. This happens when you're connecting to your spirit from your mind rather than your soul, which stems from a deep-rooted distrust of yourself. You wonder if your beliefs indeed stack up, and you're scared to be disappointed. What if your faith turns out to be fake? This idea terrifies you, Scorpio, because as someone who's naturally intuitive, you need to believe what you sense is true—otherwise, can you even trust your inner self? If you let your constant questioning get the better of you, it can cause you to second-guess the world and all that you know to be true.

But that's the ultimate test of faith. It's leaping before the net appears. It's surrendering to the unknown and believing without seeing.

When you're feeling disconnected from your spirituality, Scorpio, it's often because you're not living and acting from your spiritual truth. You're either going through the motions or grappling with doubt—or both. Get out of your mind and into your soul. Walk the spiritual path, and you'll soon see others following you.

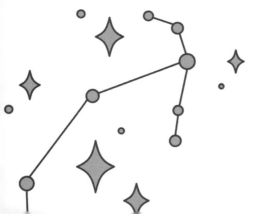

SELF-CARE TOOLS
FOR SCORPIO'S SPIRITUALITY

Your Scorpio spirit needs to ground down and walk in your spiritual truth. Do that by practicing what you preach and dedicating yourself to a spiritual-based practice that reestablishes your faith.

Find your unique spiritual routine. Ritual means everything to you, Scorpio. By dedicating time to a practice that feels right to you—whether meditating or praying or lighting a candle—sticking to a routine will help boost your faith.

Explore crystals and other spiritual tools. You're more open-minded than other signs when it comes to exploring spirituality. Explore tools like crystals and tarot cards to help tap into your natural psychic abilities and allow you to test yourself to establish trust in what you know to be true.

Try various spiritual activities. To help reaffirm your faith in yourself and the world around you, seek different spiritual activities that can help you reconnect to your soul. Going on a pilgrimage, attending a Vipassana retreat, or taking a bible study class are all examples of various things you can do to put into practice what you believe.

SAGITTARIUS

THE ALTRUISTIC ARCHER

As a Sagittarius, you're on the search for a higher truth. You seek knowledge, be it through experience, schooling, or reading. You'll talk the ear off of professors and spiritual advisors to uncover their thoughts and observations. You'll engage in long discussions with friends and family, all in the hopes of figuring out the meaning of life. Your search for answers to that big question is also what drives you to explore and travel and why you refuse to sit still or settle for an ordinary life. There's something inside you that inherently knows there's more to the world than meets the eye. You feel most connected to your spirit when you're leading a cause or spearheading a project that connects you to your passions: expansion and humanity. Ruled by Jupiter, the planet of growth and expansion, it's natural for you to seek a higher consciousness for yourself and the world around you. And as a fire sign, you want to be the one who leads the charge for that change. However, what disconnects you from your soul is when you abandon action for philosophizing. To ground yourself in your

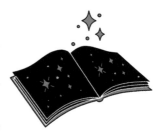

benevolent power, focus on the details of a project in order to see it through. You can be really heady at times, and your penchant for pontification comes at the price of your ability to learn more about what you preach because you're so wrapped up in the discovery of it—not the doing part of it. You might skim through books or dabble in different religions without ever diving deep into the details and understanding of what you're learning because you're so impatient about getting to the end—or receiving consciousness. However, the devil (maybe literally) is in the details and will help you further embody what you want to know. If you need help, ask for support or assistance—something you're reluctant to do. In your quest for knowledge, you also tend to be a lone wolf. You think you must disconnect from others as you try to sort out things on your own. But if you're to be someone who promotes the expansion of humanity, you need to accept the help of others sometimes and welcome them on your journey.

Allowing yourself to absorb and decipher what you're learning is how you'll reach a richer understanding of that which you seek. By welcoming the company and goodwill of others, you will ultimately possess the confidence to be a source of wisdom and be a true leader of change.

SELF-CARE TOOLS FOR
SAGITTARIUS'S SPIRITUALITY

Your Sagittarius spirit needs to welcome the assistance of others while allowing yourself to get out of your head and act on embodying your spiritual truths.

Invite others on your soul quest. Whether you're joining a new class, reading a new book, or taking a spiritual trip, invite others to join you. It will help you empathize and appreciate the help of others and learn that no person is an island. We all need each other, and being with others can enrich our lives.

Volunteer with a charity or organization. For all your good ideas on how to create change, it can be hard for you to take the necessary steps forward. Volunteering with a charity will fulfill your soul while helping you do some good in the world.

Sit outside in nature and observe. You are either moving, traveling, exploring, or immersing yourself in deep thought. Just being with yourself, quieting the mind, and observing the world around you are some of the most powerful and spiritual experiences you can have.

CAPRICORN

THE CONSCIENTIOUS AND CONSCIOUSNESS-SEEKING SEA GOAT

For someone as practical and skeptical as you, Capricorn, you're open to exploring spirituality—but on your terms. As symbolized by the Sea Goat, you're a mystic rooted in traditionalism. Your dual nature can cause some discomfort and dichotomy in your life when you don't take the time to regularly check into your spirit. If you're disconnected from your soul, you'll let the Goat side of you lead 24/7. As the logical high achiever of the zodiac, you're dedicated to working hard for your success. Ruled by Saturn, the planet of structure and traditions, you have intense boundaries and a strong sense of what you think is right and wrong. Coupled with your innate stubbornness and an old-school perspective, it's easy for you to get caught up in rigidity and pride. If you've committed to a certain way of thinking and being, even if there's a part of you that is willing to shift and get curious about something new, your ego tends to immediately shut down and continue to do what you've always done. In short: you hate change, and you hate to admit you're wrong.

However, it's important to remember that you're not a mountain goat—you're a Sea Goat. There's something special and otherworldly about you, Cap. You create your own reality alongside an inner knowingness that you're destined for more, and this knowingness stems from a belief that extends beyond the logical. When you stop leading with your mind and instead surrender to your soul, you access a divine path leading to where you're meant to be. When you can drop into this faith, you realize that you needn't be alone or try so hard on your journey. You might be the king or queen of self-mastery, but the truth is that you're a co-creator of your reality. Spirituality can be a great source of education and knowledge—which you love—while also being a sense of comfort that helps bring you closer to yourself. You don't have total control of your journey, and that can be exciting.

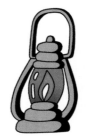

SELF-CARE TOOLS FOR CAPRICORN'S SPIRITUALITY

You need to tap into spirituality on your own terms to allow yourself to believe in your own divinity and that you're connected to a greater force that you can lean on when needed.

Dive deep into spiritual truths. You love reading and educating yourself about different perspectives and history. Understanding tenets of religion and spirituality (maybe by taking a religious history class or reading a spiritual book that's out of your comfort zone) gives you a sense of how to construct a belief system, which is what you need. Connecting your mind with your soul makes sense to you; you just need a pathway to get there.

Spend time solo. Capricorns need alone time to recharge and reset, and spending solo time helps you connect to what it means to be you. Solo time is your spiritual time, which can be as deep as asking yourself big, existential questions or as simple as reading a book in the park.

Make spirituality your own. You tend to play by the rules, but connecting to your soul and spirituality isn't a practice you need to abide by; it's something you create. Make your spirituality your own, whether that's creating a morning routine, journaling to your higher self, or connecting to a goddess circle. Get creative and dare to change it up.

AQUARIUS

CREATING A NEW FUTURE OF CONSCIOUSNESS

Y ou're a humanitarian, Aquarius, and your mission in life is to help others in the best way you can. With the Water Bearer as your symbol, you innately want to bring the masses together to help us realize just how connected and worthy we all are. While you're more tuned in to your soul and spirit than most zodiac signs, you become unbalanced when you lead with a "It's my way or the highway" mentality—ironic given how passionate you are about unity.

You are a visionary, Aquarius, so you're typically very clear on what you want to accomplish and how you want to do it. As an air sign, you're intellectualizing and brainstorming nonstop. However, you can become so headstrong about what you want to pursue that no matter how earnest and true your intentions might be, your push for progress can develop into a battle of right versus wrong ("right" being your opinion and "wrong" being anyone's opinion that isn't yours). The beauty of your mind, Aquarius, is how forward-thinking it is and how much you believe in the power of transformation and change. But you can be so focused on the future and, therefore, the idea of what *could be* that you fail to realize just how crucial the power of the present moment is. You might even become so stubborn that you detach from others involved. It becomes more about "you" than "us" or 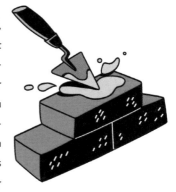 "we." Working with what you have, including who is around you, will get you further than you care to admit. Old ideas aren't necessarily bad ideas. It's important for you to realize that something new can be created on the bricks from the past; you don't necessarily need an entirely clean slate to bring about the change you wish to make. Connecting to your spirit includes learning about what was done before so you can use the best and discard the rest.

You're called to serve, Aquarius, and you're more than up to the task. While your individualism and intelligence give you a unique life perspective that can promote a revolution, your spirit must be guided by both your mind and your heart. Leaning into the community and allowing yourself to get personal with your cause will fill your cup and deliver results more than you know. Cohesion and inclusion are how you reach true consciousness.

SELF-CARE TOOLS FOR AQUARIUS'S SPIRITUALITY

Your spirit, Aquarius, needs to remain visionary. You need to feel like you're creating change while also taking time to connect and honor the good deeds of the past and those around you.

Read different spiritual and historical texts. While you usually gravitate toward technology and any books rooted in future-based thinking, reading different historical and spiritual texts will provide you with insight on the past to better inform your ideas and thinking, which, as an air sign, you will love.

Connect through a cause. You're naturally a fighter of social injustice. Volunteering and working for a cause that you're passionate about will not only fulfill you but will also connect you with a like-minded community of people from whom you can learn and with whom you can connect. Your soul and heart will thank you.

Practice yoga. Yoga is a perfect way for you to experience your spirit. It challenges your mind—which you love—while also rooting down in your body, which you often ignore. Being present with each pose and breath instantly connects you with your soul.

PISCES

~~~~~~~~~~~~~~

A FISH OF FAITH

You are the most spiritual sign of the zodiac, Pisces. You are ruled by Neptune, the planet of dreams, inspiration, and spirituality. Connecting to your soul is your natural sixth sense. You are the spiritual guru of your tribe and will gladly ponder life's meaning and your connection to it all the livelong day. You believe we're on earth for a reason and that it's your life's work to figure it out. As symbolized by the entwined Fish, representing the conscious with the unconscious, you feel like it's your duty to connect humanity with their divinity—aka a higher consciousness. You have vision boards and journal your thoughts and prayers daily. You meditate with crystals and carry a rosary. You are that friend who goes deep into spiritual texts and truths. So the irony about you, Pisces, is that you disconnect from your soul when you disconnect from yourself as a human being. You would rather indulge in your visions and undergo intense spiritual experiences than, say, do something more grounded like taking a walk in the park with a friend or helping at a soup kitchen or animal shelter. Essentially, you avoid putting your divine essence into action. But that's when you come alive as a human, Pisces. By spreading your compassionate, big heart and helpfulness to others, you show how powerful the intentions and actions of one person can be. When you turn your attention from esoteric questioning into an inner knowingness and a confidence in your capabilities to create positive change in the world, then you know what it means to be a spirit having a human experience bringing divine love to the masses.

SELF-CARE TOOLS FOR PISCES'S SPIRITUALITY

Your Pisces spirit needs to be grounded and of service in order to share your divine essence and love with the physical world.

Volunteer at a charity close to your heart. Volunteering for an organization is a perfect way to connect to your soul and your humanity, Pisces. As a natural helper and healer, you will shine by volunteering at a soup kitchen or animal shelter, which brings you into direct contact with those you are serving.

Commit to regular acts of service in your community. Your caring nature loves to help others. Committing to regular acts of service—whether mowing a lawn for a neighbor, babysitting your friend's kids, or preparing home-cooked meals for a sick family member—allows you to put your grace into action.

Tell someone you're grateful for them. No doubt you have a gratitude journal filled with adoring messages for the people you love. Let your inner circle know how you feel about them by openly acknowledging and appreciating them. When you're feeling grateful for someone, shoot them a text or send a sweet email or note to let them know.

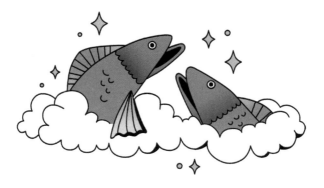

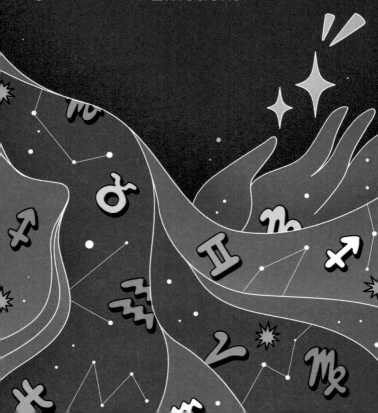

PART 5

MOOD
Embracing Your
Emotions

ARIES

SHARPNESS OVER SOFTNESS

Expressing emotions doesn't come easily to you, Aries. You like to feel in control and that you can handle everything and anything. More importantly, you're committed to doing everything by yourself. While you do feel happiest when you're running the show, sometimes your militant approach to tasks, work, and even relationships masks your immense vulnerability. The truth is that you feel a lot, Aries, but you resist opening up to others in fear of showing weakness. You despise looking weak. You believe that if others see you as fragile, they'll either be able to take away what you've worked so hard for or they'll be capable of hurting you far deeper than you care to imagine—or both.

So when something doesn't go according to your plan or a friend hurts your feelings, you're prone to lash out. Your planetary ruler, Mars, the ruler of aggression, coupled with your fire sign, makes it easy for you to lean on the feeling of rage when things don't go your way or when you feel personally attacked. You're famous for your sharp temper, and friends know to avoid

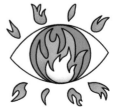

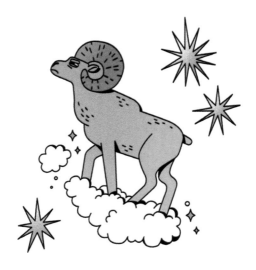

you when you're in the throes of it. You see anger as your protector despite the fact that, underneath the aggressive armor, you're really hurting inside. Without a healthy emotional outlet, your hotheadedness can cost you relationships, opportunities, and even work.

At your most vulnerable self, Aries, you have an intense fear of being forgotten or left out. That's why you initiate reunions, outings, and projects. You long for community, but you don't trust that others will include you in their plans, so you take it upon yourself to make things happen. If you do feel like a friend has slighted you, you'll either throw a fit or retreat, because that's the other side of you, Aries. When you're not seething, you shut down. You retreat into your fortress when you feel the emotions are too much to bear. You fight with yourself over feeling good enough, and instead of reaching out for support or communicating what you need or how you feel, you keep your loved ones at arm's length and disappear for a while.

Your biggest lesson when it comes to coping with emotional self-care is realizing that you don't have to go it alone. By leaning back and letting others help you, whether it's through delegating tasks for a project or allowing someone else to plan events, you're building your trust muscles and seeing the beauty and strength in teamwork and letting go. When you share your innermost feelings with a loved one and ask for support instead of shutting down, you release your pent-up emotions in a healthy way and allow yourself to connect more deeply with your loved ones, helping them to understand you better and helping you to know that you're truly accepted for being you no matter what.

SELF-CARE HABITS FOR ARIES'S FEELS

Your emotional self-care, Aries, relies on your ability to self-regulate your intense emotions while also allowing yourself to open up to your inner circle and lean on them for support.

Feeling upset? Text a friend. While your go-to might be to seethe in silence, opening up to a friend about what's bothering you and asking for their support—whether it's to help cheer you up or to ask them to take the reins for the next hangout—will take a load off your shoulders while deepening your bond with your BFF.

Take a breath. When you're feeling triggered and wanting to lash out, focusing on your breathing will help regulate your nervous system. The benefits of breathwork are threefold: it immediately brings a sense of calm to your body, it helps your mind to focus and clear, and it helps you to refrain from acting impulsively, bringing awareness to the present moment and helping your intense emotions to subside.

Move your body. You're all about physical activity, and luckily one of the best things you can do to quell anger fast is to move. Instead of throwing a fit, throw an uppercut at a punching bag or hit the mat for some yoga. Exercise stops stress and frustration dead in their tracks.

TAURUS

~~~~~~~~~~~~~~~~

AVOIDANCE AND
PASSIVE AGGRESSION

Your ruling planet, Venus, instills within you the gift of connection, which is why you're so awesome at creating and cultivating lifelong friendships and relationships. Sweet natured and compassionate, you will go the extra mile for those you care about, and your inner circle appreciates that about you. Because you take loyalty and stability seriously, you often struggle with insecurity when you feel like your friendship isn't being reciprocated. When you're not feeling balanced, it's easy for you to become hurt over simple mishaps, like an ignored text. Your anxiety is likely to skyrocket, and your mind will spin with worry over what you've done wrong. Same for any problem at work. You're one of the hardest workers of the zodiac, Taurus, so you're tough on yourself when you receive the slightest criticism from the boss. On the outside, you're a pillar of strength with a stiff upper lip, but on the inside, you're as creamy as an Oreo center.

While your sign might be a fierce Bull, the reality is you hate conflict and will avoid confrontation at all costs. You long for peace and don't like to stir the pot, which could lead you to suppressing your true feelings and voicing your opinion. As a result, you can become passive aggressive and shut out those around you. Becoming detached from the world and disappearing into your safe, cozy cocoon when you feel overwhelmed is one of your go-tos, Taurus. While taking time and space is important to process feelings, shutting down from those who care about you can cause feelings of alienation, resentment, and loneliness. And while you still might ache for connection, your stubbornness can often get the better of you, Taurus. Once you've resolved to be alone and hurt, you'll stew in those feelings for as long as possible. Without a healthy release, you can often live in denial and avoid resolving issues. As a result, you're likely to hold grudges against others and would rather endure a wall of silence than reach out to another, especially if you feel slighted.

On the flip side, if provoked, you're true to form and embody a raging Bull. You lose your temper and say things that you might later regret. However, some of these arguments could have been avoided, Taurus, had you only believed that speaking your truth is more than enough or, more importantly, that *you* are enough.

When you feel overwhelmed with the world, you second-guess your place in it and begin questioning your worthiness and value. You remain motionless and instead treat online shopping as your side hustle while drowning your sorrows in a pint of ice cream in order to fill a void.

When it comes to your emotional self-care, Taurus, it would help you to understand that you're valuable just as you are. You're a gifted creator and friend, and your presence and know-how are welcomed and admired. It is safe for you to express your feelings and needs to those around you. You are far more powerful than you realize, and it serves you to channel your emotions into something productive rather than suppress them.

SELF-CARE HABITS FOR
TAURUS'S FEELS

Your emotional self-care, Taurus, relies on your ability to express tough emotions while also allowing yourself to show up and cope with life's problems rather than run away from them.

Honor and express your emotions. What do you need to say, Taurus? It's essential to learn to honor and express your emotions no matter how difficult it might be. Talk them out with a trusted friend, advisor, or therapist. By giving an outlet to your feelings, you learn how to express them more readily when you need to. Soon you'll start to realize that talking about your feelings and addressing them in conflict isn't so hard after all.

Do something creative. Thanks to your ruling planet, Venus, you're a natural-born artist. You thrive when you're working on something that gets your creative juices flowing. This is important to remember when you're emotionally flooded. Rather than distract yourself with creature comfort like food and movies, immerse yourself with a new creative project. Draw, write, dance. It doesn't matter what you create—just follow your curiosity. Creative activities are known to instill confidence and help you authentically connect with yourself and others.

Go out in nature. Instead of retreating to your couch when emotionally triggered, head outdoors. As an earth sign, you feel naturally refreshed whenever you spend time with Mother Nature. Maybe that means popping a spot and eating lunch on a patch of grass or going on a quiet walk for a midday jaunt. Being out in nature is known to give your mind and emotions a break from being overstimulated, which means a brisk walk will leave you feeling rejuvenated and refocused.

GEMINI

SARCASTIC AND SELF-CENTERED

When it comes to emotions, Gemini, you're the Chandler of your friend group. You hide your feelings underneath a mask of good humor and offer sarcastic comments in lieu of vulnerable advice. Emotions can make you feel uncomfortable. This can cause you to come across as unsympathetic and unfeeling. However, nothing could be further from the truth. Behind your jokes and bravado lies a deep-feeling soul. You're so busy keeping everyone happy and entertained, but you secretly long to be taken care of and truly seen for all of you—including both halves of you: the half that loves bringing joy to others and the other half that longs to be emotionally honest with those around you. Underneath your goofy personality lies an amazing, loving heart, and you care deeply about those closest to you. As an air sign, though, vulnerability doesn't come easy to you, as you tend to rationalize and compartmentalize feelings. But you're human, Gemini. As much as you try to justify that logic outweighs emotions, you can't help but feel what you feel. Learning to not only accept and embrace those feelings, Gemini, but to express them softly is how you first tend to your emotional self-care.

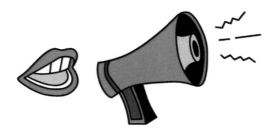

"Softly" is key, twin, because when you don't look after your own emotions, you can easily become frustrated with those around you. You turn into crankypants and tend to spew off-the-cuff remarks when you feel someone isn't on your level. The thing is, Gemini, you are two different people even at the best of times. So when you don't bring emotional intelligence into your everyday interactions, you tend to rely on the unsavory rather than the sweet side of you. You become irritable and self-centered. This is often a projection of yourself, because if you don't routinely practice self-compassion, how can you empathize with others? When in conflict, you become unreasonable and must have your own way and the last word at all costs. Your childish need to be right comes out in full force, and you refuse to acknowledge any accountability or wrongdoing. You shut down and refuse to make amends unless the other person waves their white flag first.

For you, emotional self-care is learning how to be gentle with admitting and expressing your vulnerability so that, in turn, you're able to show up fully as the compassionate person you truly are.

SELF-CARE HABITS FOR GEMINI'S FEELS

For your emotional self-care, Gemini, you're called to prioritize your feelings rather than focus on the mind, including learning more about what triggers you and why as well as learning to be with yourself.

Sit with your feelings. Vulnerability is the driving force of forming connections with others and with ourselves. Being able to reveal your feelings and desires to other people means recognizing that it's okay to feel big feelings. Don't be quick to dismiss or rationalize your feelings. Instead, sit with them and acknowledge them, and most of all, allow yourself to feel what you're feeling without judgment. Dare to be uncomfortable, and see what growth and information are coming up for you. Then extend yourself a big dose of self-compassion for who you are.

Learn about your triggers. When you're emotionally triggered, Gemini, you can be brash and push people away. Understanding your triggers is an important part of emotional self-care, as you're able to determine what irritates you or causes you anxiety. When you're triggered, take a moment to figure out why and notice if there's a pattern. Jot down what comes up; from there, you can consciously learn to navigate and manage your impulses.

Take space when feeling upset. Learning to take space to gather your thoughts, especially when you're feeling annoyed, is a great way to collect yourself and calm down. By taking space, whether it's going for a walk or going into the next room, you're able to gain more clarity about the situation, refrain from hurting others, and return to a feeling of peace.

CANCER

INSECURE AND OVERWHELMED

You abide by the rule "Mia casa e sua casa," which says a lot about the kind of loving and welcoming soul you are, Cancer. You're quick to take care of loved ones and their needs before yourself. From this place of overgiving, you often forget to fill up your own tank first. While you have a generous soul and big heart, when you're not tending to your emotional self-care, you can also be clingy and possessive of your friends. Your insecurity can override your sense of self and eventually can cause you to feel unbalanced and confused as to who you are and what you need to feel happy and healthy.

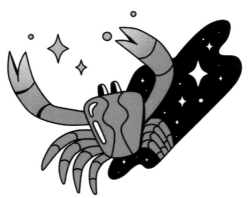

Thanks to your double whammy of emotions, courtesy of the water element and the moon that rules your sign, you are already someone who lives and breathes complex emotions. When you don't take time to learn more about what makes you tick, your emotions can become overwhelming and you struggle to process them. You become sullen and moody and retreat into your hard shell. While you yearn for the connection that vulnerability creates, you often feel unsafe to do so. You're scared of being rejected and abandoned if you reveal the truth of who you are. You might fear that you're "too much" for others to accept and embrace.

This explains why you're often passive aggressive when it comes to conflict. You'd rather suppress your feelings and carry on as if nothing were wrong in order to keep the peace. While your forgiving nature is admirable at times, it's important for you to voice your pent-up frustrations and hurt feelings so you can remain true to your values and ensure your suppressed feelings don't turn into grudges, which they often can.

If anyone can hold on to the past, Cancer, it's you. When your emotions are out of balance, you are all about nostalgia. You will ruminate and relive the past over and over again. It's difficult for you to let go of past transgressions and disappointments, so much so that it can prevent you from moving forward and living in the present moment.

As someone who lives in your emotions, it's difficult for you to detach from people and events that affected you in some way. This can lead you into experiencing a vicious loop of traumatic events without ever breaking free from them and a refusal to acknowledge the lessons and gifts that they brought into your life.

When it comes to your emotional self-care, Cancer, you must nurture yourself the same way that you nurture others. It's important for you to stand on your own two feet and claim sovereignty over your emotions. By learning to voice what you're thinking and implementing stronger boundaries with how you spend your energy, you will be better equipped to not only stay in the present moment but to enjoy it.

SELF-CARE HABITS FOR CANCER'S FEELS

Give yourself permission to talk about your feelings. Identifying what you're feeling and learning to communicate those feelings to others will help keep your emotions balanced while also allowing you to become more vulnerable so you don't have to handle tough emotions alone. Start with pausing to label what you're feeling and practicing "I feel . . ." with a trusted friend or family member.

Learn to be assertive and set boundaries. Learning to be assertive is a great lifelong lesson for you, Crab, so you can protect your own energy, handle conflict effectively, and take charge of your emotions by setting safe boundaries. Get clear on what you need to feel safe, and then name your limits on what is and isn't acceptable both for yourself and others.

Let go of the past. Getting out of your head and moving your focus from "what was" to "what is" will help you stay grounded and help you create more of what you want right now. Practice forgiving yourself and those who hurt you. Remain in the present by focusing on your breath and repeating mantras: "I forgive those who have hurt me and allow myself to move on," "I accept that my experiences are part of life's great journey, and everything I go through is to help me become the best version of myself," and "I release the pain from my heart and embrace a new beginning."

LEO

When it comes to dealing with emotions, Leo, you struggle when it comes to self-love and self-approval. This might come as a surprise to others because you're definitely someone who enjoys preening themselves and pumping your own tires. But when you're not feeling truly complete within, you crave flattery and attention to feel good about yourself. You might end up in one-way relationships in which you risk losing your identity as you become absorbed into your lover's life in an attempt to experience acceptance. You can also get caught up in a cycle of constant social comparison to others, seeking approval through "likes" and other external accolades to feel validated. As a result, you second-guess and criticize yourself for all of the things you haven't yet accomplished or acquired.

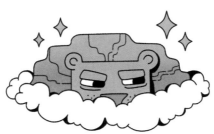

On the extreme end of the emotional spectrum, if there isn't a story to share or a situation for you to shine in, you will create drama either by embellishing some truths or spilling the tea. Of course, this is dangerous territory because you risk being called out or, worse, causing trouble for others. But when you're in this sort of "take no prisoners" frame of mind, you're not afraid of confrontation. Your growl is just as terrifying as your bite. You're short-tempered and won't back down until you win the fight—or, at least, until you feel gratified with the result, which typically means someone (not you) is licking their wounds.

Needless to say, your emotions are huge. You definitely wear the crown of Drama Queen or King when you're not feeling balanced. When you're upset or in a bad mood, everyone knows it. You think your emotions are more important than others', and if you're in the midst of an emotional meltdown, you'll make everything and anything about you. Even if a friend calls and needs your support and advice, you'll twist the conversation back to you so that you're the one who's receiving the TLC.

When you're acting like this, it's easy—and accurate—for people to accuse you of being self-centered. What you're actually craving, though, is love and understanding. However, when it comes to emotional self-care, Leo, one of your biggest lessons is learning how to facilitate confidence and self-love from within. It's important for you to learn how to soothe yourself while creating strong boundaries concerning where and how you seek acceptance. When you learn how to better balance your emotions, you'll also learn how to be a better friend.

SELF-CARE HABITS FOR LEO'S FEELS

It's important for you to learn how to self-soothe when you're experiencing big emotions, Leo, and how to be a support system for your loved ones and set boundaries with your social media.

Learn to comfort yourself. When your emotions become too big, instead of imposing them onto loved ones who might not be able to help you, take charge of your feelings by self-regulating and self-soothing. Make yourself a comforting cup of tea, scream into a pillow, and/or distract yourself with a funny movie. You can also repeat affirmations like "With each breath, I breathe in healing. With each breath, I feel calmer, more relaxed, more self-confident," "I love myself for who I am," and "I don't have to be perfect—no one is."

Take a break from social media. Take regular daily breaks from social media to help cease FOMO and any trigger—for instance, not getting a like for your latest post—that makes you feel invalid or disapproved of. Consider taking regular social media detoxes by logging out for a week every month or so.

Shine the light on others. To help practice selflessness and connect with your natural kind heart, shine the light on others. Take the backseat on a project, celebrate your friend's success, and practice active listening when a friend calls to vent. The important part of this is to be there for your loved ones and not make it about you.

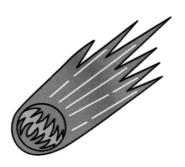

VIRGO

~~~~~~~~~~~~~~~~~~~~~~~~~~~~~~~

STOIC MEETS SANCTIMONIOUS

When you're experiencing an imbalance with your emotional equilibrium, Virgo, you can become hypervigilant with your criticism. For all your good intentions, your constant need to give advice can come across as harsh and sanctimonious. You might want someone to be the best you know they can be, but being a know-it-all only causes alienation among your close circle and can create resentment for all involved. Your feelings could get hurt if your friends dismiss your advice.

While you're typically big on communication, when you're not feeling your best, you might hold back on how you truly feel. It can be hard to talk about your feelings, even with close friends. You see emotions as information and not something to wallow in, certainly not to express. However, when you're not taking good care of your feelings, your emotional go-to is sarcasm, and you don't hesitate to throw out a caustic remark or two.

While you typically shy away from confrontation and are a peacemaker, Virgo, if you believe you've been wronged, you're not afraid to argue your case. You will fight

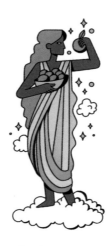

with someone until you've been proven right—even at the expense of a relationship. You'll toss out acidic sarcasm without thinking twice about how it will affect the other person as long as it validates your stance. Another classic Virgo move: you will always need to get the last word in. You do this because you need to be right—you find confidence when you have all the correct answers. The truth is, Virgo, the need to be right comes from shame in being wrong and attaching your value to being right at all costs.

In low times, as a naturally independent person, Virgo, you need your space. However, this can be to your detriment, as you tend to shut out people and convince yourself that you don't need anyone. You think problems can be solved with your intellect and mind. You choose to be stoic rather than soft. One of your biggest lessons in emotional self-care is learning to honor your emotions. If you allow that to be a freeing experience for you, it will connect you to another part of yourself that you often ignore—your heart center. Emotions are to be experienced and expressed, too—it's what makes us human.

When it comes to nurturing your emotions, Virgo, it's key to acknowledge that you have them in the first place. Accept all facets of yourself, including what you believe to be your flaws. When you begin to make self-love a priority through expressing your heartfelt truths, you'll find a more balanced way to handle the inner workings of your heart and what makes you human.

SELF-CARE HABITS FOR VIRGO'S FEELS

When it comes to your emotional TLC, Virgo, it's essential to create time and space to express and feel your emotions.

Honor and give space to your emotions. It's important for you to digest and feel what you're feeling rather than analyzing or brushing over your emotions. Carve out an hour or two each week to just be with yourself. See if there's any emotional residue that wants to move through you. Allow it come out through tears or rage. Don't judge it or label it. Just feel it.

Learn to lean on others and communicate openly. Embrace your vulnerability. Practice asking for help and support when you feel upset or need an extra hand. Smile at a new acquaintance and ask them out for a coffee. If you need space, that's okay. Instead of shutting out your inner circle, lovingly inform your loved ones that you need space and you'll get back to them when you feel better.

Let yourself and others off the hook. At the core of your need to be right and your self-righteousness is a deep fear of being wrong and making mistakes. Let yourself and others off the hook by practicing self-love and forgiveness. Compassionately accept that you're human and that being wrong and making mistakes are a part of who we are. See it as a part of growth, and continually return to loving yourself.

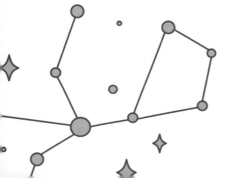

LIBRA

~~~~~~~~~~

EXPERT PEOPLE-PLEASER
AND GHOSTER

While you're naturally loving, kind, and a popular person—thanks to the planet Venus—there is an aloofness about you, Libra. You flit from social group to social group, stacking your calendar with various activities so that you keep your social status intact while keeping the vibe light and fun. You know a lot of people—but do you really know them? And do they really know the real you? Your symbol of the Scales, combined with you being an air sign, keeps you in your head a lot. When you don't honor your emotional self-care, you intellectualize emotional interactions, and it's difficult for you to openly express your vulnerability. When you're not engaged with your feelings, you skate on the surface of life and view feelings as an extension outside of yourself. They're there, but they're not fully yours. It's as if you go through the motions of emotions without actually allowing yourself to feel them.

This explains why, as much as you desire a deeper connection with others, you fear exposing your underbelly. You don't trust that others will accept you, flaws and all. Your generous

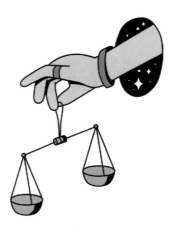

nature can stem from insecurity and cause you to bend over backward for others in order to win their approval and love. You might find yourself losing your identity in friendships and relationships and immersing yourself in their interests and lives rather than carving a life of your own. When you're not balanced and loving yourself, Libra, people-pleasing becomes your knee-jerk reaction, and you'll often go out of your way to help others rather than spending your precious time, love, and energy on you. People-pleasing is disempowering and inauthentic and leads to codependency. Pretending to be someone you're not is not only exhausting; it also robs you of expressing and owning your true self. People deserve to get to know and love the real awesome you. But mostly you deserve to celebrate and love the real you—warts and all.

Not surprisingly, as a people-pleaser, Libra, you're an expert ghoster when it comes to confrontation. Your need to keep things harmonious and in balance can teeter so far off the grid that you'd rather flee the scene at the first sight of conflict than express any discord. A naturally fickle creature, once you're done, you're done. You won't hesitate to leave a relationship at the drop of a hat without any warning. You'd rather pull an Irish goodbye than deal with hurting someone else's feelings or owning up to your side of a disagreement.

It's as if you're living life behind a mask. When you're not taking care of your feelings, you can wind up with a lot of loose ends, superficial connections, and attachments to things and people who don't align with what makes you feel good. Committing to an emotional self-care routine means connecting to your true emotions while pouring on self-compassion and love.

SELF-CARE HABITS FOR LIBRA'S FEELS

Your emotional self-care, Libra, relies on you giving yourself the space to get to know yourself: question your beliefs, dig deep into your self-love, and be your own best friend.

Give yourself some alone time. You have a hard time being alone, but solitude allows you to get to know yourself. Who are you when you're not around others? What do you like to do? What don't you like? Make a list and get curious. Then go and do those things that feel authentic to you—alone.

Reframe your assumptions on conflict. You like to think of yourself as the ultimate peacemaker, but conflict isn't all bad. In fact, conflict can be a container for growth and understanding. Fear of confrontation is often based on false assumptions. Start to assume that confrontation can be healthy and solution-oriented and not a bad thing.

Learn self-acceptance. People-pleasing comes from a fear of not being accepted. However, Libra, your own self-acceptance is worth more than anyone else's validation. Learn to love and accept yourself by writing down your achievements and all the things you like about yourself. Repeat the following mantras: "I am becoming the person I want to be. I work toward honesty and authenticity," "My decisions are my own. I stand behind my words and actions. My path is my choice," and "I can't please everyone and that's okay. I only am responsible for pleasing myself."

SCORPIO

~~~~~~~~~~~~~~~~~~

MOODY AND AGGRESSIVE SCORPION

You feel a lot of emotions, Scorpio. As a water sign, being in your feels is second nature for you. You have a lot of feelings that often oscillate throughout the day—you can be as moody as a mood ring—and when you're not grounded, they can overrun your day, confusing not only yourself but also those around you. While you definitely don't want to deny your emotions, it's important for you to find an appropriate container and/or outlet for your intense feelings. If you don't, and you've been aggravated, it's quite possible your infamous stinger will come out. When provoked, you won't hesitate to take someone down with your biting words, possibly alienating those closest to you . . . and possibly for good.

Your aggressive nature—which is a result of your planetary ruler, Mars—is typically a mask for the immense vulnerability you feel. When you're not nurturing yourself emotionally, you tend to suppress your feelings, and expressing your soft side to others is a hard no. You'll keep a cool, tough shell to keep others at arm's length, which you do to stay protected at all costs. You're terrified of being hurt or judged for your shadow; if anyone is cognizant of their shadow in the zodiac, it's you, Scorpio. You know that everyone has a good side and bad side to them—this is because of your other planetary ruler, Pluto—and when you're not nourishing your emotional self-care, you can focus too much on your flaws and faults. You might let shame overcome you, which prevents you from making connections with others.

This connection with the dark side of life can take you in two directions. Most severely, it can send you into a dark spiral of thoughts and feelings of shame and envy. When you're in this mode, you can become overly secretive and shut out others, especially if you feel slighted by a loved one. Or it can cause you to take life very seriously, making it hard for you to find the joy and light in anything. Your depth and seriousness can take over your emotional baseline, Scorpio, if you don't make time for fun and laughter.

Without a healthy emotional outlet, your emotional reactivity and serious nature can cost you relationships, experiences, and even the beauty that is life.

SELF-CARE HABITS FOR SCORPIO'S FEELS

Your emotional self-care, Scorpio, relies on your ability to self-regulate your intense emotions while also allowing yourself to open up and see the lighter side of life.

Watch something funny. Laughter sometimes is life's best medicine. Humor your funny bone and make time to watch a funny movie or TV show regularly. Even looking at a funny meme or talking to a funny friend will do the trick. Welcome the light into your life to balance the dark.

Escape to the bathtub. To help ground your emotions, go to your safe haven: water. As a water sign, you're naturally drawn to its fluid calmness. Draw a warm bath and allow yourself to sit and honor your feelings and express them however they need to be expressed. The water will soothe you and bring you back to the present.

Talk about your shadow self with trusted others. To help deepen your vulnerability and lean into your shadow self without going in a downward spiral, practice sharing your experiences with trusted friends and family. By doing so, you'll not only build a stronger relationship with yourself but also with those around you.

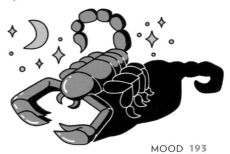

SAGITTARIUS

A BRASH AND ALIENATING ARCHER

On your best days, you have a happy-go-lucky, positive attitude that lifts spirits, Sagittarius. You have friends in many different social circles, which you love. However, sometimes your cavalier approach to relationships hides your fear of getting close to others. Your fierce independence can quickly transform into aloofness, and you're known to disappear on friends and family for periods of time to "do you." Enjoying your own company is a gift, but it's important to question why you take space from others. Is it to destress and recharge? Or is it because you're uncomfortable with getting close to others? It's usually the latter when you're not nurturing your emotional TLC. You struggle with being judged and accepted by others due to your unconventional lifestyle and views. You assume others won't "get you," so you would rather shut them out than face any criticism. It's a double-edged sword because by shutting out people before they can get close to you, you'll never know if they actually like and accept you for you— which they probably would. Much of this thinking stems from your own projection. You, too, can easily judge and criticize others, especially if you feel superior to them in any way. Because you're naturally clever and a risk taker, you take for granted the advantages you've had in life and can struggle with empathizing with others who might not be as adventurous or thought-provoking as you. As such, you either keep people at arm's length or alienate them—both of which keep you alone.

Your sharp tongue can also make your relationships tricky at times. Your brashness, while often done in the name of love and truth-telling, can sting and hurt those closest to you. You might think you're doing them a favor by cutting to the heart of the matter, but they might view you as cold and insensitive. While it would better serve you to deliver news more tactfully, when you're fired up, you can't help yourself. As a fire sign, you're impulsive and passionate, and you say and do what feels right to you in the moment.

This can also be a selfish tic of yours. After all, you're a brazen trailblazer who seeks to build new enterprises and explore new opportunities and sceneries simply because you want to. You're so busy chasing after your own dreams that you seldom stop to consider how your choices and decisions affect others. While you do care about the special people in your life, it's easy for you to put your needs and wants above others.

When it comes to coping with emotional self-care, your biggest lesson is learning that you needn't do life alone. There are people who appreciate you for you and will expect the same from you. Relationships are a two-way street. You don't have to sacrifice your independence for the right connections, but there is some goodness and joy to be had when you see life can be better with others. Compromise and cooperation can be gifts to you too if you let them.

SELF-CARE HABITS FOR SAGITTARIUS'S FEELS

Your emotional self-care, Sag, relies on your ability to empathize with others while allowing yourself to accept your flaws and accept others for theirs.

Do a judgment check-in. It's important to keep yourself in check, whether you're judging others or yourself. When you feel judgmental, ask yourself why. Notice what triggers your thoughts, whether about you or others. Stop to consider the reason for someone's behavior or perspective. If you're judging yourself, reframe your thoughts with affirmations: "My uniqueness is awesome and worth celebrating," "I am deeply loved and appreciated for who I am," and "I am unique, and my dreams and aspirations are unique to me. I do not need to prove myself to anyone."

Show care and concern. When someone's upset, chances are they want emotional support or need their feelings acknowledged. That doesn't always mean giving someone advice or serving them up a truth bomb. Before you go in for a tongue-lashing, ask them how you can help or support them. Consider their needs before yours. Regularly putting yourself in another's shoes will help you understand others and keep you connected.

Ask others to join you. You need others in your life, Sagittarius, and they need you, too. Being around others and including them in your experiences help you destress, stave off feelings of loneliness, and increase your state of happiness and sense of belonging and well-being. Have your alone time, but balance it with some scheduled social time.

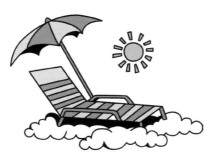

CAPRICORN

SUPPRESSED
AND SERIOUS SEA GOAT

You're often a serious and stoic Goat. You're so caught up in the busyness of your world and achieving your goals that it can be difficult for you to crack a smile. That's too bad, because underneath that measured demeanor is someone who's adept with a wry and sarcastic comment. You're funny, Capricorn! But when you're bogged down by your tasks and errands, you forget that life's not that serious. Or at least it doesn't have to be all the time. Finding your balance between letting your hair down and being true to your need for space is the sweet spot when it comes to nurturing your emotions.

Speaking of space, while it's healthy to require alone time, when you're not in a great place, it's easy for you to shut down and shut out those around you. In sticking with

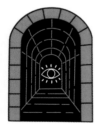 your stoic appearance, you can also be aloof to even those closest to you. You prefer to process feelings and emotions alone. Underneath your stiff upper lip is a gentle and sensitive soul who longs for belonging. But you often build a fortress

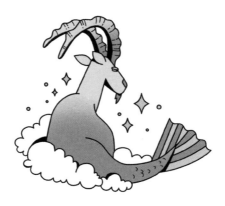

around your feelings because you're scared of caring too much. Your often intense mistrust of others causes you to worry that you'll be abandoned by those who you love the most. As a naturally shy person, it can be hard for you to open up to new people in general, so once you find your people, you're all in. You have loyalty to your friends and family like no other sign in the zodiac. Your sentimentality for your loved ones runs deep, and you're scared of being forgotten by them or, worse, dumped. So you'll push people away and hide your most vulnerable self before anyone can leave or judge you.

You definitely have a well of feelings. When you're annoyed or irritated with others, you won't hesitate to put someone in their place or start an argument. You have a quick temper and can mince people with your words. While you are open to having a grounded conversation after the fact, sometimes it can be too late. Learning how to cool your jets and recognize your triggers will save you a lot of grief and keep you balanced enough to bite your tongue or respond in a more constructive manner.

When it comes to emotional self-care, you need to acknowledge and access all of your feelings, Capricorn. By doing so, you'll be able to balance your work with play and enjoy the ones you love the most, including yourself.

SELF-CARE HABITS FOR CAPRICORN'S FEELS

Your emotional self-care, Capricorn, relies on your ability to self-regulate your intense emotions while also allowing yourself to open up to your inner circle and lean on them for support.

Feel your feelings. You have a ton of repressed feelings, Cap. Expressing yourself is a safe way for you to let them out and realize just how normal and healthy it is to experience a range of emotions. Cry, scream, or laugh. Do whatever you need to connect to how you really feel.

Talk it out with a friend. You're someone who often thinks sharing emotions is a sign of weakness. However, being vulnerable with those you trust the most is a fantastic way to process your feelings and to form deeper bonds. Vulnerability is the glue that keeps relationships strong.

Connect to your funny bone. Connecting to and reveling in your joy is key for you, Cap, because you tend to veer toward work and stoicism. But you have a wicked sense of humor and can easily entertain others when you let your hair down. Get silly! Watch funny movies and TV shows and experiment with telling jokes to friends. Try an improv or standup comedy class. Indulge in fun!

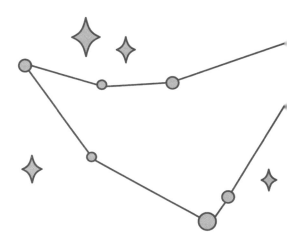

AQUARIUS

DISCONNECTED AND INDIFFERENT

As friendly and altruistic as you are, Aquarius, you tend to come off as cold, indifferent, and aloof to even your closest friends. You're a loner by nature and like your space, but when you're not nurturing your emotions, you can be even more impersonal toward those around you. As an air sign, you're more disconnected from your feels, preferring to lead with logic and a sense of fair judgment. Emotions are messy and cause attachments, and you like to stay as detached and drama-free as possible.

Deep down, you have a distrust of emotions; as a result, you keep people at arm's length. This can confuse and hurt your inner circle. Your planetary ruler, Uranus, gives you a need for freedom and an ingrained fear of losing control. You're secretly scared to be vulnerable, which links to a fear of rejection and abandonment. You march to the beat of your own drum, and you're well aware that you come across as a

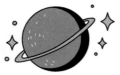 little "out there" at times. It's hard for you to fit in sometimes, which can make you feel insecure and lead you into a spiral of self-judgment and shame. Like everyone,

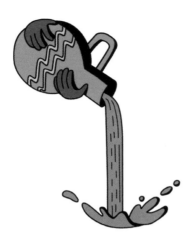

you just want to be loved as is. But when you keep people away and shut off your truest emotions, you don't allow others the opportunity to get to know and love the real you.

You don't abide by the "once bitten, twice shy" thinking. Once bitten, and you're outta there, no second tries. While you're naturally a peacemaker and will try to find the most logical and reasonable resolution to a conflict, you can easily hold a grudge if you're wounded by a loved one. Cutting someone out of your life is easy for you. Denying someone's emotional hold on you is your forte. You convince yourself that you don't "need" anyone.

You're independent, a deep thinker, and super analytical, Aquarius, which serves you well when you're diving into your latest project and cause. You also have a lighter side that doesn't get to come out as much when you're lacking in the emotional self-care department. You tend to withdraw and ruminate when things get heavy, but sometimes laughter really is the best medicine—and you have a wicked sense of humor that your friends really enjoy.

When it comes to emotional self-care, allow yourself to experience your feelings full-on and see the beauty of connection. Happiness can be found in light and laughter and the company of others.

SELF-CARE HABITS FOR AQUARIUS'S FEELS

Your emotional self-care, Aquarius, relies on trusting others to love and honor you and to do the same for yourself.

Schedule some one-on-one time with a friend. It's easy for you to get caught up in your own stuff and keep your friends on the backburner. Schedule regular one-on-one hangouts with your friends so you can maintain and grow your connections while also making time to have thoughtful and vulnerable conversations. It will remind you how fun and comfortable it is to share time with a trusted loved one.

Make some time to LOL. Don't forget that you need to lighten your mood! Tap into your natural sarcastic side by watching funny movies, going to comedy clubs, calling a funny friend, and sharing funny GIFs. When you find yourself brooding, reach for the funny to shake things up.

Ask for space and help before you need it. Your urge to flee is rooted in anxiety and fear. When your stressors keep coming and you refuse to address them, your need to withdraw due to burnout and insecurity becomes real AF. Let your loved ones know what's going on with you before you bolt. It will help them understand you better and give them the opportunity to help you. Take the support sometimes— it's okay to let people help you.

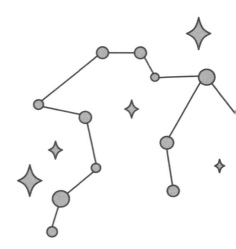

PISCES

~~~~~~~~~~~~~~~~~~~~~~~~

AN OVERLY EMOTIONAL AND
DESPONDENT FISH

Expressing emotions is second nature to you, Pisces. As an emotional and intuitive water sign, you're basically a walking and talking beating heart. You feel and absorb everything from everyone. You're an extreme empath, which makes it difficult for you to determine which feelings are yours and which belong to others. When you're not taking the time to nurture your emotional self-care, you're vulnerable to developing depression, anxiety, and emotional burnout. You can become so despondent that doing anything and going anywhere becomes almost impossible. You'd rather shut yourself off from the world than engage in it. You isolate yourself from friends and family and can fall into a deep emotional spiral.

Being so empathetic also makes you susceptible to attracting narcissists at one extreme or becoming a people-pleaser at the lighter end of the spectrum. You're already naturally accommodating and flexible, Pisces, but when you're not taking care of your own emotional well-being, you put others' needs before your own. It's not out of character for you to drop everything to be at a friend's or lover's beck and call. You might tell yourself that you're being compassionate and doing it out of love, but if you're not acting from your integrity, chances are you're acting out of insecurity and a fear of not being loved in return. While it's a beautiful thing to be the sage counselor and healer of your inner circle, it's important that you allow yourself to receive that TLC—from others and yourself.

However, you're not so much of a pushover that you fail to realize when you're being scorned or taken advantage of. When this happens or any other conflict occurs, you have no trouble throwing a tantrum and making a play for the Best Actress Oscar. When it comes to your taste for theatrics, you keep your emotions at one hundred. While you don't particularly enjoy conflict—in fact, you'll avoid it as much as possible to keep the peace—you have difficulty

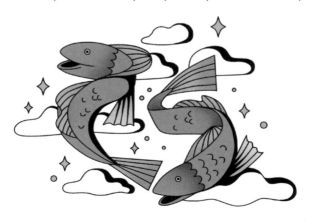

controlling your emotions at times and can easily make a mountain out of a molehill, which might alienate you from others. You might try your best to soothe their feelings, as you often do, but if you've decided you're done, you have no trouble ghosting them. No surprise—confrontation isn't exactly your strong suit.

When it comes to coping with emotional self-care, your biggest lesson is learning how to control your emotions rather than be controlled by them. Your empathic nature is a beautiful gift but only when you're able to learn to honor your abilities with confidence and self-love. By grounding yourself and navigating your sensitivity, you're able to finally put yourself first so you can ultimately serve others.

SELF-CARE HABITS FOR PISCES'S FEELS

Your emotional self-care, Pisces, relies on your ability to self-regulate your intense emotions so they allow you to live your best life.

Come back to your body. When you're emotionally flooded or feeling extra sensitive, ground yourself into your body and into the present moment. Wiggling your toes and caressing your wrists slowly while actively relaxing any tension in your body with five big exhales will calm your sensory and nervous systems and keep you centered.

Detox in water. As a Pisces, you love being in water, and a great way to dissolve stress and emotional overload is by detoxing in a warm Epsom salt bath with magnesium. Add a little lavender essential oil to calm your nerves, and visualize your intense feelings dissolving in the tub.

Learn to set boundaries. Boundaries are your friend, Pisces. Learning to set limits with people will keep you from feeling drained or like a doormat and will help you better communicate with others. It's okay not to go to your friend's party if you don't feel like it. If someone is yelling at you, it's okay to tell them you don't want to further engage until they've calmed down. "No" is a complete sentence, and saying it regularly will empower you.

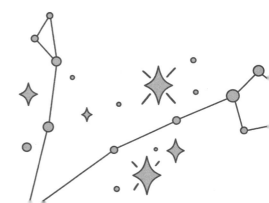

PART 6

YOUR
SELF-CARE
ROUTINE
CHECKLIST

When you're feeling unbalanced or just need a quick reference for self-care, take a look at your zodiac self-care checklist below.

THE ARIES SELF-CARE ROUTINE CHECKLIST

☐ Recite affirmations: "When I allow myself to slow down, I can be my badass self," "Rest is productive, too," and "My worth is determined by who I am and not by what I do."

☐ Work out! Check out the latest HIIT class or go to a volleyball meet-up.

☐ Fill your schedule with activities you actually want to do. Include some volunteer work that appeals to your soul.

☐ Take the time to do breathwork during the day—especially when you're feeling overwhelmed.

☐ Have something weighing on your mind? Text a friend and talk to them about it!

- ☐ If you're feeling disconnected from the world around you, ask yourself what small act of kindness you can do for someone else today.

- ☐ Go for a walking meditation after work to calm the nervous system and reconnect to self.

- ☐ Don't forget downtime! Read a chapter of a fun book or watch a favorite show to wind down after dinner.

- ☐ Still feeling awake and/or stressed? Practice yoga before bedtime.

THE TAURUS SELF-CARE ROUTINE CHECKLIST

- ☐ Regularly do something out of your comfort zone. It can be as simple as taking a different route to work or ordering a new type of salad for lunch.

- ☐ When you have a long to-do list, commit to tackling one goal at a time. Recruit an accountability buddy, and don't forget to reward yourself for a job well done!

☐ Are you upset about something? Call a trusted friend or book an appointment with your therapist to let it all out.

☐ Organize! What are you holding on to that you no longer need? Does your closet need to be cleaned out?

☐ Create something, especially if you're feeling emotionally flooded.

☐ What are you thinking about that is no longer serving you? Don't forget your affirmations: "I take charge and get things done right now," "I am always supported by life no matter what," and "I believe in myself and my capabilities."

☐ Move your body daily. Take a walk in the park or go swimming! Do something that feels good.

☐ Cook something new and healthy, then eat it mindfully.

☐ Take the time to walk outdoors. Not only will it ground you, but it's also a perfect form of exercise for you.

☐ Before bed, write down five things for which you are thankful in your gratitude journal.

THE GEMINI SELF-CARE
ROUTINE CHECKLIST

☐ Create a morning routine so that you feel organized and grounded to start off the day. This is a great way to be alone with your thoughts as you sip your coffee and journal your feelings.

☐ Practice mindfulness throughout the day to stay present and focused.

☐ Plan your meals for the week to ensure you're eating balanced and healthfully.

☐ Take yourself out on weekly solo artist dates where you tackle new creative activities, like visiting an art gallery or a dance class.

☐ Attend your team sport league night, or call your personal trainer to schedule a sweat session.

☐ Feeling emotional? Instead of pushing away your feelings, take some time to sit with them and acknowledge why they're coming up.

☐ Before bed, make a list of everything you appreciate in your life, especially the small things.

THE CANCER SELF-CARE ROUTINE CHECKLIST

☐ Make a plan. Whether it's your daily to-do list or a business outline, create a plan for your goals to keep you focused and clear.

☐ Commit to doing something that pulls you out of your comfort zone, like speaking to a stranger at the bank or trying a new hobby.

☐ Do something creative, especially if you're suppressing a lot of emotions.

☐ Feeling upset? Call or text a friend to talk about what's bothering you, and implement some boundaries if needed.

☐ Commit to exercise—maybe it's a home workout or something connected to the water.

- [ ] Cook at least one plant-based meal this week, and skip dessert until the weekend.

- [ ] Connect to your intuition by journaling and starting a lunar meditation practice.

- [ ] Volunteer your time with a charity where you can connect to others.

- [ ] Having trouble letting go of the past and struggling with embracing the new? Don't forget your mantras: "I forgive those who have hurt me and allow myself to move on," "I accept that my experiences are part of life's great journey, and everything I go through helps me become the best version of myself," and "I release the pain from my heart and embrace a new beginning."

THE LEO SELF-CARE ROUTINE CHECKLIST

- [ ] To connect with spirit and your expressive nature, take some time to chant in the morning.

- [ ] Before your confidence takes a hit, create a humble-brag file of your greatest achievements.

☐ Don't forget you're a natural artist and you need to create for the sake of creativity! Book some time to paint or dance or whatever feels good to you.

☐ When you want to take more control of things you can't control or fall victim to the compare game, refer to your fear list—what are you really afraid of? Get clear on the root of the issue to release it.

☐ Feeling overwhelmed by your emotions? Remember your affirmations: "With each breath, I breathe in healing. With each breath, I feel calmer, more relaxed, more self-confident," "I love myself for who I am," and "I don't have to be perfect; no one is."

☐ Get your body moving with a fun group workout or a team sport.

☐ When you look at yourself in the mirror, don't forget to give props for your body and all that it can do for you.

☐ Shine the light on others—whether it's cheering on a friend's new business venture, donating your time anonymously, or paying for a stranger's coffee.

☐ When a friend calls, listen actively and focus on them and the support they need.

☐ Take a social media break. Don't check your social media before bed. Instead, focus on you and what makes you feel good about yourself.

THE VIRGO SELF-CARE ROUTINE CHECKLIST

☐ Create a morning spirituality practice such as reading a sacred text or delving deeper into spiritual truths and knowledge.

☐ Feeling overwhelmed? Visualize what you want to happen and what can go right instead of what could go wrong.

☐ Still feeling anxious? Lean on others and communicate openly to those around you, whether asking for help or sharing your feelings.

☐ If you don't feel like sharing feelings with others, make space for your emotions so you don't blanket them with reason and logic.

☐ Laugh at yourself more. When you're feeling overly critical of yourself, take a minute to laugh at your circumstances—life isn't so serious all the time. Read a funny meme or watch a funny movie to break the tension.

☐ Take a day off. You need to rest and recharge your busy mind. Implement a rest day that's truly relaxing, including a day when you don't work out. Instead, indulge your senses and appetite.

☐ Go for a hike. Being outside grounds you, and hiking is a pleasant way to move your body. While you're outside, take the time to meditate outdoors for 15 minutes.

☐ Do some Zen yoga after work to connect your mind and body for the ultimate workout that will both relax and energize you.

☐ Return to self-love by repeating these affirmations: "My worth isn't based on my achievements," "I am exactly where I am supposed to be, and I am doing exactly what I am supposed to be doing," and "Today will be what it is. I will be who I am. And there will be beauty in both."

THE LIBRA SELF-CARE ROUTINE CHECKLIST

☐ Ease a fearful mind by meditating for at least 15 minutes. Then, connect with your spirit with freewriting.

☐ Struggling to make a decision? Think back to when you made a good decision. What did you do? Drop out of your busy mind and listen to your body. What feels right to you? Trust your instincts.

☐ Challenge your fear-based thinking. If you were to do something—or not—what would really happen? Challenge your fears and flip the script.

☐ Give yourself some alone time to get in touch with who you are. Make a list of things you enjoy doing, then go do them—alone.

☐ Don't forget to squeeze in a workout: try a team sport or a Barre or Pilates class.

☐ Assign a sweet day to moderately balance your sweet tooth.

☐ In conflict? Ease your anxiety by reframing your assumptions about how bad it can be, and practice voicing your true feelings.

☐ Attend a religious or spiritual service to connect with those in the community to feel the oneness of all.

☐ Learn to love and accept yourself by writing down your achievements and what you love about yourself. Repeat the affirmations: "I am becoming the person I want to be. I work toward honesty and authenticity," "My decisions are my own. I stand behind my words and actions. My path is my choice," and "I can't please everyone, and that's okay. I am responsible for pleasing only myself."

THE SCORPIO SELF-CARE ROUTINE CHECKLIST

☐ Start your day with your spiritual ritual. Tap into your intuition with crystals or tarot cards.

☐ Take consistent action on one goal.

- [ ] Stumped with an idea or not knowing how to move forward? Brainstorm all sorts of positive outcomes and ideas to offer more flexibility.

- [ ] Move your body with a run, Kundalini yoga, or a Zumba class.

- [ ] Take a load off and watch something funny to lift your mood.

- [ ] Look for spiritual getaways you might want to take to reconnect with yourself.

- [ ] If you find yourself falling deep in thought and going dark, remember your uniqueness. Consider opening up to a friend.

- [ ] Unwind in the bathtub and have a private moment with yourself to find your center.

THE SAGITTARIUS SELF-CARE ROUTINE CHECKLIST

~~~~~~~~~~~~~~~~~~~~~~~~~~~

☐ When you feel judgment kicking in, ask yourself where it's coming from. If you feel especially self-critical, reframe your thoughts: "My uniqueness is awesome and worth celebrating," "I am deeply loved and appreciated for who I am," and "I am unique, and my dreams and aspirations are unique to me. I do not need to prove myself to anyone."

☐ Create consistency by sticking to a bedtime and morning routine.

☐ Feeling stifled? Do some creative visualization to calm your nervous system and to visualize new possibilities for yourself.

☐ If you're suffering from wanderlust, start planning your next trip, or try learning a new language or a new cuisine.

☐ Schedule workouts that are intense and varied like HIIT and boxing, or head outdoors for trail running.

☐ Ask others to join you in a new activity, whether it's a new spiritual experience or a new hobby.

- [ ] Before dropping a truth bomb on a friend, stop and put yourself in their shoes. Consider what their needs are and how you can best support them.

- [ ] Volunteer for a charity or organization to stay connected to others and a good cause.

- [ ] Do you feel overwhelmed? Make it a rest day. Consider going outdoors and observing the scenery in silence for at least 15 minutes.

THE CAPRICORN SELF-CARE ROUTINE CHECKLIST

~~~~~~~~~~~~~~~~~~~~

- [ ] Surrender the things you can't control. Consider a positive outcome. Recite: "I don't need to sweat the small stuff," "I let go and trust the outcome," and "I trust the process of life."

- [ ] Feeling overwhelmed and anxious? Get out of your head and reconnect with your body by taking a quick walk around the block or stretch at your desk.

- ☐ Allow yourself to be messy and make a mistake. Don't complete your to-do list or worry about wearing the fanciest clothes.

- ☐ Make time to make yourself and others laugh.

- ☐ Schedule a workout session that's challenging and gets you outside, like mountain climbing or trail running.

- ☐ If you're feeling in your feels, express them or talk it out with a friend.

- ☐ Spend some time alone to connect to yourself and be totally present with yourself.

- ☐ Create a spiritual practice that's only yours, whether it's reading history and texts, meditating, or praying.

- ☐ At night, journal your feelings to examine and express them.

THE AQUARIUS SELF-CARE
ROUTINE CHECKLIST

☐ Plan and prep your meals for the week, whether that's cooking or picking out the healthiest takeout options.

☐ Feeling burned out and ready to flee? Let your friends and family know how you're feeling so they can offer you support—or at least know where you're at.

☐ If you're feeling cagey and distracted, breathe and remind yourself: "I believe in who I am," "No matter what I am journeying toward, the fullest expression of my truth is a valuable road to be on," and "My unique-ness is worth celebrating because it brings something special to the world."

☐ Make some time in your day to LOL, whether it's with a funny TV show, movie, or meme.

☐ Create! Get out of your logical mind by painting, brainstorming, dancing, or doing anything that allows you to see things from a fluid perspective.

- ☐ Schedule some quality time with a friend to catch up—and don't forget to share your feelings.

- ☐ Volunteer with a cause that you're passionate about.

- ☐ Exercise! Check out your fitness app or sign up for a karate class. Practice some yoga to bring some calm, and connect with your spirit afterward.

- ☐ Before bed, read a spiritual text and write in your gratitude journal to further connect to your soul and help you see all that you have right here and now.

THE PISCES SELF-CARE ROUTINE CHECKLIST

- ☐ Start your day off with a plan of action. What are you creating this week? Tell a friend to stay accountable. Repeat affirmations: "I take full responsibility for my life so that I may live my dreams," "Every action I take moves me closer to my dreams," and "I have faith in myself and my abilities."

☐ Feeling distracted on a project? Take a moment to look around at your surroundings and play the A–Z game to stay focused.

☐ Schedule some fitness time, either with a swim, dance class, or jog with your accountability partner.

☐ Feeling emotionally flooded? Take five big exhales, wiggle your toes, and caress your wrists to ground yourself.

☐ Channel your creative side with a new class! Painting, pottery, cooking. What are you interested in?

☐ Ensure you're setting boundaries with those in your life. Is your friend incessantly texting you all day? Tell her that you'll get back to her when you have a moment, and silence your phone.

☐ Commit to acts of service, whether through helping in your community or at a local charity.

☐ Tell a loved one how much you appreciate them in a sweet text.

☐ Unwind at the end of the day with a warm Epsom salt bath to dissolve any icky feelings.

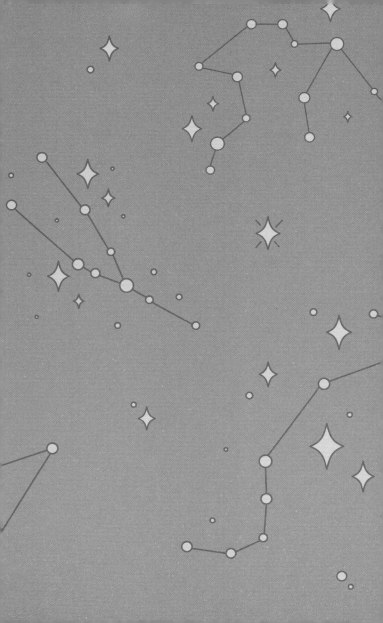

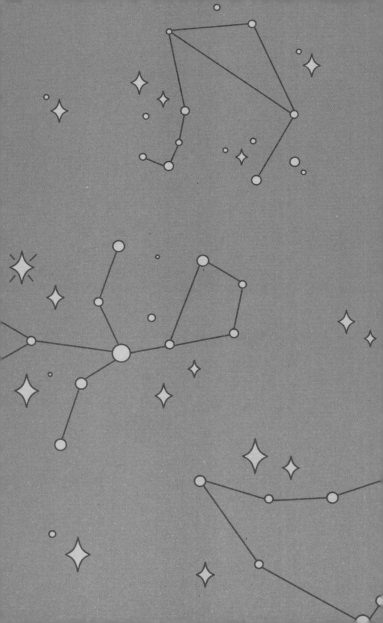